disha
Nurturing Ambitions

Errorless

AF519236

NCERT SOLUTIONS with 100% Reasoning for Class 12 BIOLOGY

• **Corporate Office :** 45, 2nd Floor, Maharishi Dayanand Marg, Corner Market, Malviya Nagar, New Delhi-110017

Tel. : 011-49842349 / 49842350

By :
Sanju Priyadarshi
Anshu Narula

Typeset by Disha DTP Team

DISHA PUBLICATION

ALL RIGHTS RESERVED

© Copyright Publisher

No part of this publication may be reproduced in any form without prior permission of the publisher. The author and the publisher do not take any legal responsibility for any errors or misrepresentations that might have crept in. We have tried and made our best efforts to provide accurate up-to-date information in this book.

For further information about the books from DISHA,

Log on to **www.dishapublication.com** or email to **info@dishapublication.com**

Contents

Preface

NCERT Books are one of the **most important resources for every student preparing for his/her school board examination. It also forms the basic foundation for competitive examinations like PMT, JEE, NTSE, Olympiad** etc. The Exercises at the end of each chapter or In-chapter not only captures the essence of the whole chapter but also helps in understanding the various kinds of questions that can be asked in the examination. Thus understanding explanations of these questions builds your confidence and interest in the subject.

The book '**Errorless NCERT Solutions with 100% Reasoning Class 12 Biology'** is exclusively written to provide best quality solutions to all the Questions/ Exercises given after every chapter/ In-chapter.

The **Unique Selling Point of this book** lies in the following:

- **Chapter at a glance,** provides crisps points which will help the students to revise their NCERT chapter.
- **100% Errorless Reasoning** (which is missing in Most of the Books), explain step-by-step to bring 100% Concept Clarity for the student and help them to write the solution in board exam according to marking scheme. The solutions are Complete (each and every question is solved), Inflow (exactly on the flow of questions in the NCERT book) and Errorless.
- **Notes,** which is given immediately after the solutions provides Important Tips, extra information (which is helpful to solve questions of competitive level), Alternative Methods, Points to Remember etc.

Although we have taken utmost care while preparing this book. But still some errors might have crept in, we hereby request our readers to report them at the email id given below. This will help us in our endeavour to create 100% AUTHENTIC & ERRORLESS SOLUTIONS TO NCERT BOOKS.

All the Best........

Disha Team

feedback@aiets.co.in

Chapter 1

REPRODUCTION IN ORGANISMS

CHAPTER AT A GLANCE

- The period from birth to death is known as **life span**. The life span of the organisms varies from one organism to another organism.
- Life span depends upon the juvenility, maturity (stage when one starts to reproduce), ageing and senescence, and death.
- **Reproduction** is a biological process in which an organism gives rise to young ones similar to itself. It allows and ensures the species continuity generation after generation.
- Living organisms reproduce by three different modes of reproduction:
  (i) Asexual reproduction
  (ii) Vegetative reproduction
  (iii) Sexual reproduction

ASEXUAL REPRODUCTION

- **Asexual reproduction** is a process of producing individuals whose genes come from single parent only with the help of mitotic division.
- Offsprings produced are genetically and morphologically similar to each other and to the parent, hence they are also called as **clones**.
- Asexually reproducing organisms reproduce faster than sexually reproducing organisms.
- The biggest disadvantage of asexual reproduction is absence of diversity.
- Asexual reproduction occurs most commonly in unicellular organisms, in plants and in certain animals that have relatively simple organisations.
- Asexual reproduction takes place by following methods: binary fission; multiple fission; budding and spore formation, vegetative propagation.
- In **binary fission** a cell simply copies its DNA and then splits in two, giving a copy of its DNA to each daughter cell. For example, bacteria and archaebacteria.
- **Multiple fission** is a process in which the nucleus of the parent cell divides several times by amitosis, producing several nuclei. It occurs in many protists, e.g. sporozoans and algae.
- **Budding** is a process in which a new organism grows off the side of the parent through a part (called a **bud**, which means small growth). Bud detaches itself to form a new organism. Budding can occur both in unicellular and multicellular organisms. For example, bacteria yeast, protozoan, *Hydra*, etc.

- In **spore formation**, the parent body produce numerous spores (within a sac-like structure called sporangium) which can produce new plants. It is surrounded by a hard-protective cover to withstand unfavourable conditions like high temperature and low humidity. Under favourable conditions, the spores germinate and grow into new plants. Moss, fern, molds and mushroom reproduce by using this method. The most common of these structures are zoospores.
- In **fragmentation**, a "parent" organism is split into multiple parts, each of which grows to become a complete, independent "offspring" organism. This process resembles budding and vegetative propagation, but with some differences.
- **Vegetative propagation** occurs in plants. In plants, the units of vegetative propagation like runner, rhizome, sucker, tuber, bulb are called vegetative propagules. All are capable of producing new offsprings.
- The **main advantage of vegetative propagation methods** is that the new plants contain the genetic material of only one parent, so they are essentially clones of the parent plant. This can also help to maintain consistent quality and taste in products made from plants or crops.
- Examples of vegetative propagules are rhizome of ginger, eyes of potato, bulbil of agave, leaf buds of *Bryophyllum*, sucker in apple and banana, offset of water hyacinth.

SEXUAL REPRODUCTION

- Sexual reproduction involves the fusion of male and female gametes. It results in offspring that are not identical to the parents or to themselves.
- When male and female gametes are produced from male and female parents respectively, then it is called **unisexual reproduction**, e.g., man, cow, etc.
- When both male and female gametes are produced from same individual, then it is called **bisexual reproduction**, e.g., earthworm, tapeworm.
- **Events in sexual reproduction can be grouped into three distinct stages:** pre-fertilisation events, fertilisation and post-fertilisation events.

Pre-fertilisation events

- Pre-fertilisation comprise all the events of sexual reproduction which takes place before the fusion of gametes. There are two main pre-fertilisation events-gametogenesis and gamete transfer.
- **Gametogenesis** is the process of formation of two types of gametes through meiosis. Gametes (male or female) are haploid cells.
- Gametes are of **two types:**
  - **Homogametes (also called isogametes)** are morphologically similar in appearance and not categorised into male and female gametes. For example, algae (*Cladophora*).
  - **Heterogametes** are morphologically two unique female and male gametes. For example, antherozoid or sperm is the male gamete and egg or ovum is the female gamete.

- Plant may be **bisexual** (containing both malc and female reproductive structure on same plant) or **unisexual** (containing male and female reproductive structure on different plant).
- In some plants and fungi, bisexual condition is also called as **homothallic** (or **monoecious**) and unisexual condition is called as **heterothallic** (or **dioecious** condition).
- The unisexual male flower is **staminate**, i.e., bearing stamens, while the female flower is **pistillate** *i.e.* bearing pistils.
- In some flowering plants, if both male and female flowers may be present on the same individual or on separate individuals are respectively called as **monoecious** (e.g, cucurbits and coconuts) or **dioceous** (e.g., papaya and date palm).
- Most animals are dioecious, for example, insects, spiders, fish, amphibians, reptilians, birds and mammals. They all exhibit **sexual dimorphism**.
- **Hermaphroditism** is a condition of having both male and female reproductive organs.
- **Gametic transfer**
  - Gamete transfer is a process in which gametes are bring together to facilitate its fusion or the process of fertilisation.
  - In most of the cases, male gamete is motile (algae, bryophytes & pteridophytes) and the female gamete is stationary except for few fungi and algae in which both types of gametes are motile.
  - In seed plants, pollen grains are the carriers of male gametes and ovule has the egg or female gamete. Pollen grains produced in the anthers are transferred to the stigma by a process, known as **pollination**.
  - Pollination is of **two types:** self pollination and cross pollination.
  - **Self pollination** is the process of transfer of pollen grains from anther to stigma occurs within the same flower, e.g., pea.
  - **Cross-pollination** is the process of transfer of pollen grains from anthers of male flower to the stigma of female flower of different flowers through the agency of air, water or animals particularly insects.

Fertilisation (also called **syngamy**)

- It is the complete and permanent fusion of two gametes from different or same parent to form a diploid zygote.
- It may be external or internal on the basis of place of fusion of gametes.
- In **external fertilisation**, parents release sperms and eggs into the surrounding water, where fertilisation takes place and zygotes develop into offspring, e.g., *Obelia*, *Nereis*, *Labeo* and Frog.
- **Internal fertilisation** is characterised by sperm fertilising the egg within the female. Internal fertilisation protects the fertilised egg or embryo from predation and harsh environments, which results in higher survival rates than can occur with external fertilisation.

- There are some organisms in which the female gamete undergoes development to form new organisms without fertilisation. This process is known as **parthenogenesis**, e.g., rotifers, honeybees and some lizards.

Post-fertilisation events

- After the formation of zygote, it develops into an embryo & the process is known as **embryogenesis**.
- During embryogenesis, a new individual is formed by the process of cell division and differentiation.
- **On the basis of a development of zygote**, the animals are of two types: oviparous and viviparous.
- The **oviparous animals** lay fertilised or unfertilised eggs. For example, reptiles & birds.

  The **viviparous animals** give birth to young ones. For example – majority of mammals, including humans.
- In flowering plants, the zygote is formed inside the ovule of the ovary.
- The **ovary develops into fruit** which develops a thick wall called **pericarp** that is protective in function. Under favourable condition, seeds germinate to produce new plants.

EXERCISE

1. Why is reproduction essential for organisms?

Sol. Reproduction, as the characteristic feature of all living organisms, is the ability to produce a young one similar to itself.

It is *essential for organism* because it helps in survival and ensures the continuance of various species on the earth. In its absence the species will not be able to exist for a long time and may soon get disappeared from the earth.

2. Which is a better mode of reproduction: sexual or asexual? Why?

Sol.
- Sexual reproduction is a *better mode of reproduction as compared to asexual reproduction.*
- It is because of the following reasons:
  - Asexual reproduction allows very little or no variation throughout their generation, due to which the individuals produced are exact copies of their parents and themselves.
  - Sexual reproduction allows the formation of new variants by combining DNA of two different parents. The offspring produced from the fusion of male and female gamete are not identical to their parents and to themselves. Due to such variation, the individuals constantly adapts the changing and challenging environment for their survival and leads to the evolution of better suited organisms which ensures the greater survival of a species.

Note

The variation that sexual reproduction creates among offspring is very important to the survival and reproduction of the population.

3. Why is the offspring formed by asexual reproduction referred to as clone?

Sol. Asexual reproduction is a type of reproduction in which a single individual is capable of producing offspring without involving fusion of male and female gametes.

Offspring produced by asexual reproduction is referred to as clones because clone are genetically and morphologically similar and the offspring produced by asexual reproduction are not only genetically and morphologically similar to one another but also similar to their parent.

4. Offspring formed due to sexual reproduction have better chances of survival. Why? Is this statement always true?

Sol.
- *Yes, the offspring produced by sexual reproduction have better chance of survival* because they are not only genetically identical to their parents but also exhibit variations which lead them to adapt the changing environment for their better survival. Asexually produced organisms are genetically identical and all organism show similar adaptations. So, during any calamity, there is a possibility that the whole generation would destroyed leading to extinction of species.
- However, the given statement – "*the offsprings produced due to sexual reproduction has better chance of survival" is not always true* because of the following reasons –
  (i) There are some inborn genetic disorders due to which organism have a risk in their survival, e.g., haemophilia.
  (ii) Asexual reproduction is a fast and a quick mode of reproduction which does not consume much time and energy as compared to sexual reproduction.

5. How does the progeny formed from asexual reproduction differ from those formed by sexual reproduction?

Sol. The progeny formed from asexual reproduction differ from those formed by sexual reproduction because, in asexual reproduction offspring (progeny) is produced by a single parent without the formation and fusion of gametes and involves only mitotic cell division that gives rise the daughter cells which are genetically identical to the parent cell. It does not show any variation among offsprings hence called as clones. Whereas, in sexual reproduction offspring is produced by two parents. It involves meiotic cell divisions producing haploid nuclei which on fusion produce offspring that are genetically different from their parents.

Organism thus produced show variation from each other and their parents.

6. Distinguish between asexual and sexual reproduction. Why is vegetative reproduction also considered as a type of asexual reproduction?

Sol. • The difference between asexual and sexual reproduction are as follows :

S. No.	Asexual reproduction	Sexual reproduction
1.	It occurs only in invertebrates and lower chordates.	It occurs almost in all types of animals.
2.	It is always uniparental and does not involve fusion of male and female gametes.	It is usually biparental and involves the fusion of male and female gamete.
3.	Gametes are not formed.	Two types of gametes are formed.
4.	It involves only mitosis.	In involves both meiosis and mitosis.
5.	Daughter organisms are genetically identical to the parent.	Daughter organisms genetically differ from their parents.
6.	Since there is no variation, so it does not contribute to evolution of the species.	Because of variations, it contributes to the evolution of species.

- *Vegetative reproduction is considered asexual reproduction* in plants because it does not involve the fusion of male & female gamete to produce new plant, rather vegetative plant parts like rhizome, runner, sucker, tuber, bulb all are capable of producing new offspring. These parts give rise to daughter individuals without the involvement of two parents.

7. What is vegetative propagation? Give two suitable examples.

Sol. • *Vegetative propagation*, a method of asexual reproduction in plants, is a process which does not involve the production of seeds or spores for the propagation of new plants. In this propagation, the vegetative parts of plants (like runners, rhizomes, suckers, tubers etc.) other than seeds are used as vegetative propagules. This method is carried out by those plants which have lost their capacity to produce seeds or produce non-viable seeds (e.g., Banana, seedless grapes, rose, pineapple, etc.)

- *Examples of vegetative propagation:*

  (i) Underground modified stems such as rhizomes (e.g., Ginger, *Eichhornia* or water hyacinth, etc.), corms (e.g., *Colocasia*, Banana, etc.), bulbs (e.g., Garlic, onion, etc.), etc. are able to give rise new offsprings. Rhizomes are root-like stems that grow horizontally under the ground. New roots and shoots form at the nodes with shoots growing upwards to form new plantlets. Lateral buds grow out to form new rhizomes.

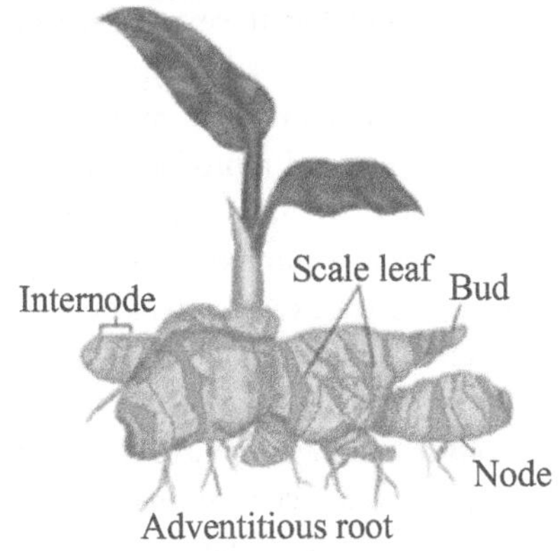

Fig.: Rhizome of ginger

(ii) Vegetative propagation by leaves in *Bryophyllum*, *Begonia* etc. *Bryophyllum* have adventitious buds coming out from the notches of the leaves. In these plants, plantlets develop from the buds present on the marginal notches of the intact leaves. These plantlets become detached and develop into independent plants.

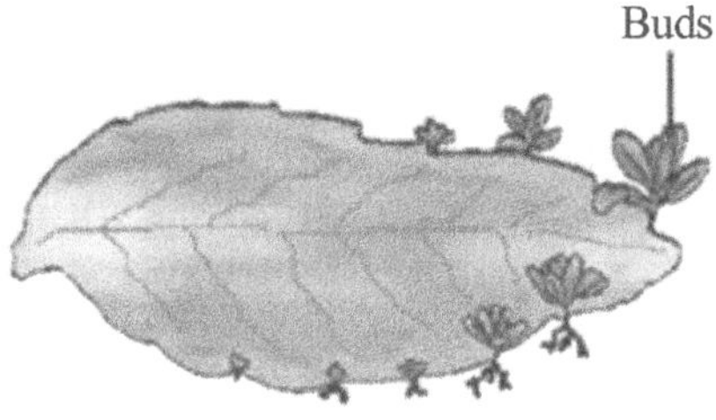

Fig.: Leaf of *Bryophyllum* with buds

8. Define :

(a) Juvenile phase

(b) Reproductive phase

(c) Senescent phase.

Sol. (a) Juvenile phase : All organisms have to reach a certain stage of growth and maturity in their life before they can reproduce sexually. That period of growth is called juvenile phase. However, this phase is known as vegetative phase in plants.

(b) Reproductive phase : The end of juvenile/vegetative phase marks the beginning of reproductive phase. During this phase, the organisms reproduce sexually and produce offspring.

(c) Senescent phase : It begins from the end of the reproductive phase. It is the period when an organisms grows old and lose the ability to reproduce.

9. Higher organisms have resorted to sexual reproduction in spite of its complexity. Why?

Sol. Although sexual reproduction involves more time and energy, higher organisms have resorted to sexual reproduction in spite of its complexity because sexual reproduction results in multiplication and perpetuation of species and also contributes to evolution of species by introducing variation much more faster as compare to asexual reproduction in a particular population. Sexual reproduction enables higher organisms to survive during unfavourable conditions.

10. Explain why meiosis and gametogenesis are always interlinked?

Sol.
- *Meiosis* (a process which occurs during gametogenesis, involves the reductional division in which the amount of genetic material is reduced) *and gametogenesis* (the process of the formation of gametes) are *always interlinked* because gametes produced by organisms are haploids (contaning one set of chromosomes), while the body of an organisms is diploid.
- Therefore, for producing haploid gametes (gametogenesis) the germ cells of an organisms undergoes meiosis. During the process of meiosis the meiocytes of an organisms undergoes two successive nuclear and cell divisions with a single cycle of DNA replication to form haploid gametes. Thus, gametes are formed as a result of meiosis so that their chromosome number remains constant.

11. Identify each part in a flowering plant and write whether it is haploid (n) or diploid (2n).

(a) Ovary __________________

(b) Anther __________________

(c) Egg __________________

(d) Pollen __________________

(e) Male gamete __________________

(f) Zygote __________________

Sol. (a) 2n (b) 2n (c) n (d) n
(e) n (f) 2n

12. Define external fertilisation. Mention its disadvantages.

Sol.
- When fusion of the gametes takes place outside the body of the organisms in an external medium, generally water, it is called *external fertilisation or external syngamy*. This form is found in many aquatic animals like fishes, amphibians, majority of algae. During the process, parents release eggs and sperms in the surrounding water, then fertilisation and development of offspring occur externally.
- *Disadvantages of external fertilisation*
  (i) It occurs only in aquatic medium.

(ii) A chance factor is involved requiring synchronous release of gametes nearby and absence of turbulence of water.

(iii) There is no protection to young ones which results in a low rate of survival of the progenies and are vulnerable to a number of predators.

(iv) Eggs have less chances of fertilisation. This can lead to the wastage of a large number of eggs produced during the process.

Note

Animals using external fertilisation strategy does not rely on hormones, mating rituals and behavioural factors to ensure that the male and female have sexual intercourse.

13. Differentiate between a zoospore and a zygote.

Sol.
- Zoospores are the microscopic, flagellated (motile) special asexual reproductive structures found in certain members of the kingdom fungi and simple plants like algae whereas zygote is a diploid cell formed by the fusion of male and female gametes. The zygote is usually nonflagellated.
- Zoospores are the structures that give rise to new organism whereas zygote is formed after fertilisation which develops into a mature organism.

14. Differentiate between gametogenesis from embryogenesis.

Sol. Differences between gametogenesis and embryogenesis

S. No.	Gametogenesis	Embryogenesis
1.	It is the formation of male and female gametes.	It is the formation of embryo from the zygote.
2.	Gametes are the haploid cells.	Embryo is a diploid cell.
3.	Both mitotic & meiotic cell division take place.	Only mitotic division occur.

15. Describe the post-fertilisation changes in a flower.

Sol. After fertilisation the zygote is formed. The zygote then undergoes many divisions by the process of mitosis, to form an embryo by a process called embryogenesis. In sexual reproduction, events that occur after the formation of zygote are called post-fertilisation events.

The *Post-fertilisation changes in a flower* are:

- In flowering plants, the zygote is formed inside the ovule.
- After fertilisation the sepals, petals and stamens of the flower wither and fall off. But the pistil remains attached to the plant.
- The zygote develops into the embryo and the ovules develop into the seed. The seed contains an embryo, enclosed in a protective covering, called the seed coat. As the seed grows, further, another floral parts wither and fall off. This lead to the growth of the ovary, which enlarges and ripens to become a fruit with a thick wall called the pericarp.

16. What is a bisexual flower? Collect five bisexual flowers from your neighbourhood and with the help of your teacher find out their common and scientific names.

Sol.
- Flowers in which male and female sex organs (stamens and carpels) are borne on the same flowers are called bisexual flowers.
- *Examples of plants bearing bisexual flowers* are as follows:
  (i) *Brassica* (sarson) – *Brassica campestris*
  (ii) Onion – *Allium cepa*
  (iii) Garden pea (Edible pea) – *Pisum sativum*
  (iv) Petunia – *Petunia hybrida*
  (v) *China rose* (shoe flower) – *Hibiscus rosa-sinensis.*

17. Examine a few flowers of any cucurbit plant and try to identify the staminate and pistillate flowers. Do you know any other plant that bears unisexual flowers?

Sol.
- By studying a flowering plant of family cucurbitaceous it is noted that cucurbit plant bears unisexual flowers as these flowers have either the stamen or the pistil. Male flowers are present at the summit peduncles and female flowers are solitary.
- The male or staminate flowers of cucurbits bear bright coloured petals and a prominent group of stamens. Male plants or staminate flowers do not bear fruits.
- The female or pistillate flowers bear fruits. In a fertilised young pistillate flower very small fruit is visible below petals and sepals.
- Other examples of plants that bear unisexual flowers are: Papaya, Mulberry and Date-palm.

18. Why are offspring of oviparous animals at a greater risk as compared to offspring of viviparous animals?

Sol. Animal shows different methods of production of young ones. Oviparous and viviparous are such two methods.

Offsprings of oviparous animals are at greater risk as compared to offspring of viviparous animals because,

- In oviparous animals, the development of the zygote takes place outside the body of the female parent whereas in viviparous animals, it takes place inside the body of the female.
- In oviparous animals, the fertilised eggs are laid in the open environment where they are not protected from the predators and their whole embryonic development is exposed to harmful environmental and biological factors.

Thus, the survial rate of oviparous animals is very less as compared to offspring of viviparous animals.

Chapter 2

SEXUAL REPRODUCTION IN FLOWERING PLANTS

CHAPTER AT A GLANCE

- Flowers and their parts are responsible for sexual reproduction in angiosperms.
- Fruits and seeds are the end products of sexual reproduction.
- Flowers, usually have four different kinds of floral members (*i.e.,* calyx, corolla, androecium and gynoecium) arranged in four whorls.
  - **Calyx :** It consists of number of green leafy **sepals**. It is the **outermost whorl.**
  - **Corolla :** It consists of a number of usually bright coloured **petals** and is the **second whorl in the flower**.
  - **Androecium :** This is the **male whorl** and consists of **stamens** and each stamen can be regarded as modified leaf (microsporophyll) that consists of **filament** and **anther**. The anther may contains two-four microsporangia that produce a large number of **pollen grains**.
  - **Gynoecium :** It is present in the centre of the flower and is the **female reproductive whorl**. Its unit is called **carpel**. Each carpel is made up of 3 parts — ovary, style and stigma.
- Sexual reproduction in plants is **divided into three events-** (i) Pre-fertilisation events (which includes microsporogenesis, megasporogenesis, pollination), (ii) Fertilisation and, (iii) Post-fertilisation events (which includes embryogenesis and seed formation).

PRE-FERTILISATION EVENTS

- The process of fertilisation starts much before the actual fertilisation takes place. Formation of flower and its component parts- stamen and pistil, are pre-requisite for fertilisation.
- **Microsporogenesis**
  - The process of formation of microspores or pollen grains is called **microsporogenesis**.
  - Pollen grains consist of outer "exine" and inner "intine". **Exine** is composed of sporopollenin which is resistant to physical and biological decomposition. It protects the pollens from environmental extremes. **Intine** is thin, delicate, cutin and cellulosic layer lying internal to exine.
  - Mature pollen grain contains two cells – a large, nucleated **vegetative cell** which is irregular in shape with abundant food reserve and a small spindle shape **generative cell**.
  - In most of the angiospermic species, pollen grains are shed at two-celled stage while the others shed them at three-celled stage.

- **Megasporogenesis**
  - The process of formation of megaspore from megaspore mother cell (MMC) is known as **megasporogenesis.**
  - A female gametophyte *i.e.* embryo sac consists of egg apparatus, synergids and antipodals.
  - Egg apparatus consists of two synergids and one egg cell lying at the micropylar end. Two polar nuclei form the central cell. Three cells present at the chalazal end constitute antipodals.
- **Pollination**
  - The process of transfer of pollen grains from anther to the stigma of a pistil is known as **pollination.**
  - Pollination is facilitated by various factors like wind, water, insects, birds and animals.
  - Transfer of pollen grains from anther to stigma of same flower is called **self-pollination or autogamy.**
  - Transfer of pollen grains from anther to the stigma of another flower of the same plant or genetically similar plant is called **geitonogamy**.
  - Transfer of pollens from the anther of one flower to stigma of another genetically different flower is called **cross-pollination or xenogamy**.
  - **Agents of pollination :** abiotic agents [wind (anemophily), water (hydrophily)] and biotic agents [insects (entomophily), birds (ornithophily), bats (chiropterophily), and animal (zoophily)].
  - Plants are modified variously to ensure cross-pollination by **self sterility (self-incompatibility), dichogamy, herkogamy, unisexuality, heterostyly**.
- **Pollen-pistil interaction**
  - Pollen grain germinates on the stigma to produce a pollen tube through one of the germpores on its surface.
  - If the pollen grain is released at the two celled stage (*i.e.*, vegetative and generative cells) then generative cell divides meiotically to produce two male gametes, but when pollen grain are released at 'three'-celled stage then two male gametes are already present.
- **Artificial hybridisation**
  - Artificial hybridisation is one of the major approaches of crop improvement programme. It can be achieved by emasculation and bagging.
  - Dusting of pollen from a chosen plant on to the stigma of the selected plant artificially for obtaining commercially superior varieties is called **artificial hybridisation.**
  - During antificial hybridisation, stigma is protected from pollination from unwanted pollen grains.

FERTILISATION

- Following entry of pollen tube inside one of the synergids during pollen-pistil interaction, it bursts releasing two male gametes into the cytoplasm of the synergids.
- One of the male gametes moves towards the egg cell and fuses with its nucleus to form a diploid cell, the zygote (2n). This fusion brings about the **syngamy**.

- The other male gamete fuses with two polar nuclei of the central cell to produce triploid primary endosperm cell (PEC) (3n). Since, the latter involves fusion of three haploid nucleus, therefore it is called **triple fusion**.
- In some angiosperms, two types of fusion "syngamy" (leading to the formation of zygote) and "triple fusion" (forming primary endosperm cell) occurs in same embryo sac. This phenomenon is called **double-fertilisation**.

POST-FERTILISATION EVENTS

- Following double fertilisation, post-fertilisation events involves the process of endosperm and embryo development and maturation of ovule(s) into seed(s) and ovary into fruit.
- **Endosperm** is the nutritive tissue which provides nourishment to the embryo in seed plant.
- Primary endosperm cell undergoes continuous division without being immediately followed by cell wall formation leading to the formation of a large number of nuclei. This forms a **free-nuclear endosperm**.
- In some plants, endosperms lack free nuclei stage, which are called as **cellular endosperms** (e.g., *Datura, Petunia*) and some endosperm have free nuclei which are called as **nuclear endosperms** (e.g., maize, wheat, rice etc.).
- Dicotyledonous plants have **two cotyledons** while monocotyledonous plants have only **one cotyledon**.
- **Seed** is the final product of fertilisation in angiosperm and acts as a **main propagative unit in plants**.
- Ovules mature into seed and simultaneously ovary develops into a fruit.
- **Types of seeds**
  - **Albuminous seed :** Those seeds which contains some endosperm that acts as food storage tissue. E.g., Dicots – castor, poppy, custard apple. Monocots – cereals, millets, sugarcane.
  - **Non-albuminous seed :** Those seeds that are devoid of endosperm. E.g., Dicots – gram, pea, bean, mustard, mango. Monocots – orchid, alisma.
- After fertilisation ovary begins to grow and gradually matures into fruit.
- The wall of the ovary develops into the wall of fruit called **pericarp**.
- The **fruits may** be **fleshy** as in guava, orange, and mango, or may be **dry**, as in groundnut, and mustard.
- In most plants, by the time the fruit develops, other floral parts degenerate and fall off.
- **Types of fruits**
  - **True fruit :** Normally it is a ripe ovary that grows into the true fruit, e.g., cucumber, tomato, coconut.

    False fruit : When floral parts other than ovary (particularly thalamus or even calyx) form part of the fruit, e.g., apple, cashewnut, strawberry.
  - **Parthenocarpic fruit :** In some plants, ovary may grow into fruit without fertilisation, e.g., oranges, watermelon, banana, grapes.
- **Apomixis** is the production of seed without fertilisation.
- The normal process of cell cycle involving meiosis and fertilisation is called **amphimixis**.
- **Polyembryony** is the state of occurrence of more than one embryo in a seed, e.g., citrus and mango.

EXERCISE

1. Name the parts of an angiosperm flower in which development of male and female gametophytes take place.

Sol. The process of the development of male gametophyte and female gametophyte is called microgametogenesis and megagametogenesis respectively.
The *male gametophyte* or the pollen grain *develops inside the pollen chamber of the anther*, whereas the *female gametophyte* (also known as the embryo sac) *develops inside the nucellus of the ovule* from the functional megaspore.

2. Differentiate between microsporogenesis and megasporogenesis. Which type of cell division occurs during these events? Name the structures formed at the end of these two events.

Sol. • Differences between microsporogenesis and megasporogenesis

S. No.	Microsporogenesis	Megasporogenesis
1.	It is the process of formation and differentiation of pollen grains (or microspores) from diploid microspore mother cells by meiosis.	It is the process of formation and differentiation of haploid megaspores from diploid megaspore mother cells by
2.	Pollen grains are produced in the microsporangium or pollen sac of an anther which is a broader knob like fertile part of the stamen.	It occurs inside the megasporangium or ovules of seed plants.
3.	All the four pollen grain that are formed from microspore mother cell are functional.	Only one out of the four megaspores is functional, while other gets degenerated.

- *Meiosis* occurs in both the events of microsporogenesis and megasporogenesis. Process of meiosis or reduction division results in the formation of haploid gametes from the microspore and megaspore mother cells.
  Each microspore mother cell and megaspore mother cell contain two sets of chromosomes and are therefore diploid. The diploid megaspore mother cell and microspore mother cell enlarges and undergo meiosis to produce, four haploid cells called megaspores and microspores respectively. The chromosome number is reduced by half and therefore megaspores and microspores are haploid.
- At the end of these two events, *microsporogenesis and megasporogenesis give rise to pollen grains and embryo sac respectively*. Pollen grain is the male gametophyte and embryo sac represents the female gametophyte.

3. Arrange the following terms in the correct developmental sequence : Pollen grain, sporogenous tissue, microspore tetrad, pollen mother cell, male gametes.

Sol. The *correct developmental sequence* is as follows:

Sporogenous tissue – Pollen mother cell – Microspore tetrad – Pollen grains– Male gametes.

During the development of microsporangium, each cell of the sporogenous tissue acts as a pollen mother cell and gives rise to a microspore tetrad, containing four haploid microspores by the process of meiosis (microsporogenesis). As the anther matures, these microspores dissociate and develop into pollen grains. The pollen grains mature and give rise to male gametes.

4. With a neat, labelled diagram, describe the parts of a typical angiosperm ovule.

Sol. A typical angiospermic ovule is a female megasporangium where the formation of megaspores takes place. It is formed in the ovary.

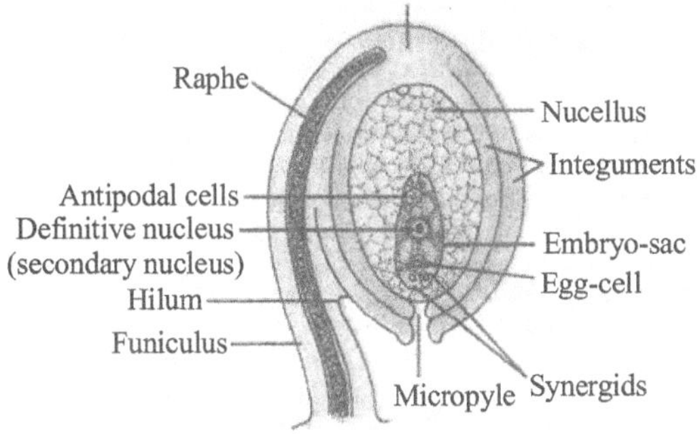

Fig.: A typical angiosperm ovule

- The *various parts of an ovule* are –
  - (i) Hilum – It is the point where the body of the ovule is attached to the funiculus.
  - (ii) Funiculus – It is a stalk-like structure which represents the point of attachment of the ovule to the placenta of the ovary.
  - (iii) Micropyle – It is small opening which is left by the integument in the ovule for the passage of pollen tube into the ovule.
  - (iv) Integuments –They are the outer layers surrounding the ovule that provide protection to the developing embryo. It forms seed coats *i.e.* testa and tegmen.
  - (v) Chalaza – It is the basal region of ovule from where the integuments arise.
  - (vi) Nucellus – It is a mass of the parenchymatous tissue surrounded by the integuments from the outside. The embryo sac is located inside the nucellus. It provides nourishment in the development of embryo sac.
  - (vii) Embryo sac – It is the female gametophyte which contains the egg apparatus, antipodal and polar nuclei.
  - (viii) Raphe – It is the longitudinal ridge formed by lengthwise fusion of funiculus with the body of ovule in a typical anatropous ovule.

Note

Angiosperm ovules are diverse in their position in the ovary, nucellus thickness, number and thickness of integuments, degree and direction of curvature, and histological differentiations.

5. What is meant by monosporic development of female gametophyte?

Sol. In many flowering plants, *monosporic development of the female gametophyte* is a process in which only one out of the four megaspores enlarges and develops into female gametophyte or embryo sac.

A single megaspore mother cell which is present at the micropylar pole of the nucellus region of the ovule in most of flowering plants undergoes meiosis to produce four haploid megaspores. Later, out of these four megaspores, only one functional megaspore develops into the female gametophyte, while the remaining three degenerates.

6. With a neat diagram explain the 7-celled, 8-nucleate nature of the female gametophyte.

Sol. Female gametophyte, commonly known as embryo sac, develops from a single functional megaspore. This megaspore undergoes three successive mitotic divisions to form eight nucleate embryo sacs.

The first mitotic division in the megaspore forms two nuclei. One nucleus moves towards the micropylar end while the other nucleus moves towards the chalazal end. Then, these nuclei divide at their respective ends and re-divide to form eight nucleate stages. As a result, there are four nuclei each at both the ends *i.e.,* at the micropylar and the chalazal end in the embryo sac. At the micropylar end, out of the four nuclei only three differentiate into two synergids and one egg cell. Together they are known as the *egg apparatus*. Similarly, at the chalazal end, three out of four nuclei differentiate as antipodal cells. The remaining two cells (of the micropylar and the chalazal end) move towards the centre and are known as the *polar nuclei*, which are situated in a large central cell.

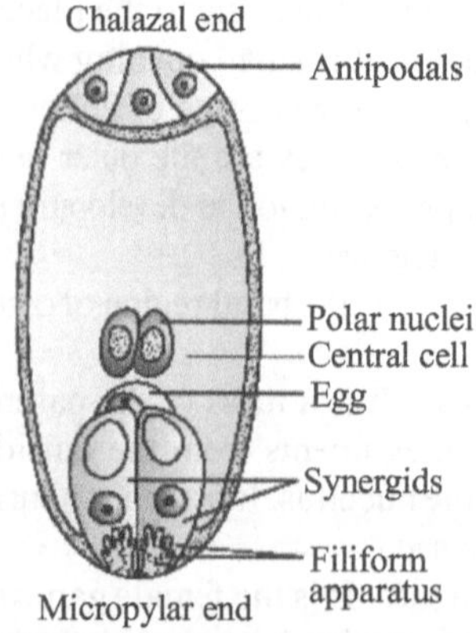

Fig.: A diagrammatic representation of the mature embryo sac

Hence, at maturity, the female gametophyte appears as a 7-celled structure (an egg, two synergids, three antipodals and a central cell), though it has 8 nucleate.

7. What are chasmogamous flowers? Can cross-pollination occur in cleistogamous flowers? Give reasons for your answer.

Sol.
- *Chasmogamous flowers* (or open flowers) are bisexual flowers in which anthers and stigmata are exposed for pollination.
- *Cross-pollination* (the process of transfer of pollen from the flower of one plant to the flower of a plant having a different genetic constitution) *cannot occur in cleistogamous flowers*, because these flowers never open at all and also, the anther and the stigma lie close to each other in these flowers. Hence, only self-pollination is possible in these flowers. Cleistogamous flowers remain in bud form throughout their life and form seeds *via* self-pollination. In such flowers, anthers dehisce inside the closed flowers. So the pollen grains come in contact with stigma. Thus, there is no chance of cross-pollination, e.g., *Oxalis, Viola*.

8. Mention two strategies evolved to prevent self-pollination in flowers.

Sol. Self-pollination is the transfer of pollen from the anthers to the stigma of the same flower or of another. It always occurs in bisexual flowers. Continued self-pollination decreases the vigour and vitality of a particular race. Thus, flowering plants have developed many devices to discourage self-pollination and to encourage cross-pollination.

- *Two strategies that have evolved to prevent self-pollination* in flowers are **dichogamy** and **self-incompatibility**.
  (i) Dichogamy is the maturation of anther and stigma at different times in a bisexual flower which prevent self-pollination.
  (ii) Self incompatibility (also called self sterility) is a genetic mechanism and prevent self-pollen (from the same flower or other flowers of the same plant) from fertilising the ovules by inhibiting pollen germination or pollen tube growth in the pistil.

9. What is self-incompatibility? Why does self-pollination not lead to seed formation in self-incompatible species?

Sol.
- When the pollen grains of an anther do not germinate on the stigma of the same flower, then such a flower is called self-sterile or incompatible and such condition is known as *self-incompatibility or self-sterility*.
  It develops genetic incompatibility between individuals of the same species or between individuals of different species. Examples are tobacco and potato.
- *Self pollination does not lead to seed formation in self incompatible species* because in self-incompatibility, the plants which exhibit this phenomenon have the ability to prevent pollen germination, pollen tube growth, ovule fertilisation or embryo development at one of its stage. This prevents the fusion of the gametes along with the development of embryo. As a result, no seed formation takes place.

10. What is bagging technique? How is it useful in a plant breeding programme?

Sol. • *Bagging* is process of covering flowers on male as well as female parents in separate bags (made up of polyethene, muslin or paper) after emasculation to prevent contamination of its stigmas with unwanted pollens.
When the stigmas of emasculated flowers mature the bags are removed, stigmas are dusted with pollen grains of desired male plants by means of a presterilised brush and flowers are rebagged till fruit develop. This technique is mainly used in artificial hybridisation.

• Bagging technique is an *important part of plant breeding programme* because,
  (i) It ensures that pollen grains of only desirable plants are used for fertilisation of the stigma to develop the desired plant variety.
  (ii) It helps to avoid inbreeding depression caused by self-pollination.
  (iii) Commercially superior hybrid varieties can be obtained by cross pollination of different useful species.

11. What is triple fusion? Where and how does it take place? Name the nuclei involved in triple fusion.

Sol. • *Triple fusion* is the fusion of second male gamete with the two polar nuclei located in the central cell to form the triploid primary endosperm nucleus (PEN). It is also called vegetative fertilisation.

• This process *takes place in the embryo sac of angiosperm.*
After reaching the ovary, pollen tube enters into the embryo sac from the micropylar end. After penetration, the tip of the pollen tube ruptures releasing the two male gametes. The one male gamete fuses with the egg to form the diploid zygote (called syngamy) and the other male gamete fuses with the two polar nuclei to form the triploid (3n) primary endosperm (called as triple fusion). These two events of fertilisation constitute the process of double fertilisation.
It results in the formation of the triploid primary endosperm cell.

• Nuclei involved in triple fusion are *two polar nuclei* and *nucleus of male gamete.*

> **Note**
>
> *Syngamy is a type of generative fertilisation whereas triple fusion is a type of vegetative fertilisation. Syngamy occurs in animals and fungi as well. But, triple fusion only occurs in angiosperms.*

12. Why do you think the zygote is dormant for sometime in a fertilised ovule?

Sol. Zygote is formed by the fusion of the male gamete with the nucleus of the egg cell. It *remains dormant for sometime in a fertilised ovule* because the outer conditions like high temperature, humidity, improper light, etc., are not favourable for germination. So therefore, it waits for the endosperm to form as it is the source of nutrition for the developing embryo. Endosperm develops from the primary endosperm cell resulting from triple fusion and provides food for the growing embryo and after the formation of the endosperm, further development of the embryo from the zygote starts.

13. Differentiate between:

(a) Hypocotyl and epicotyl

(b) Coleoptile and coleorrhiza

(c) Integument and testa

(d) Perisperm and pericarp

Sol. (a) Differences between hypocotyl and epicotyl

S.No.	Hypocotyl	Epicotyl
1.	It is the part of embryonal axis in between cotylendonary node and radicle.	It is the part of embryonal axis in between plumule and cotyledon node.
2.	In epigeal germination, hypocotyl elongates so that cotyledons come out of soil.	In hypogeal germination, epicotyl elongates so that cotyledons remain in the soil.
3.	The terminal end of hypocotyl is radicle.	The terminal end of epicotyl is plumule.

(b) Differences between coleoptile and coleorhiza

S.No.	Coleoptile	Coleorhiza
1.	The epicotyl bearing shoot apex and leaf primordia is enclosed in a foliar structure called coleoptile.	The radical and root cap are enclosed in a sheath called coleorhiza .
2.	Coleoptile has a terminal pore for the emergence of first leaf.	Coleorhiza is a solid structure.
3.	It protects the plumule during emergence from soil.	It does not protect the radicle during its passage
4.	It grows much beyond the grain.	After emergence from grain it stops growing.
5.	Coleoptile after emergence from soil during germination, becomes green (due to presence of chlorophyll) and does photosynthesis.	Coleorhiza does not come out of soil. It remains nongreen end is pale in colour.

Note

Similarities between coleoptile and coleorhiza: *These are structures of the monocot seed. Both act as a protective sheath. Also, both undergo rapid growth in its early phase.*

Difference between coleoptile and coleorhiza : *Coleoptile is the sheath that protects the emerging shoot while coleorhiza is the sheath which protects the emerging root.*

(c) Differences between integument and testa

S.No.	Integument	Testa
1.	It is the covering of the ovule.	It is the outer covering of seed.
2.	It is thin, one or two layered.	It is quite thick and one layered.
3.	Its cells are living.	Its cells are dead.
4.	Sclereids are absent.	Cells are rich in sclereids.
5.	It arises from chalazal end of ovule.	It is derived from outer integument of ovule after fertilisation.
6.	It is pre-fertilised structure.	It is a post-fertilised structure.

(d) Differences between perisperm and pericarp

S.No.	Perisperm	Pericarp
1.	It is unused nucellus in the seed.	It is the covering of fruit that develops from ovary wall.
2.	It is a part of seed.	It is a part of fruit.
3.	It is usually dry.	It is dry or fleshy.
4.	It is often non-functional for seed.	It is protective covering and also helps in dispersal and nutrition.
5.	It is present in only a few seeds such as beat and black pepper.	It is found in all fruits.

14. Why is apple called a false fruit? Which part(s) of the flower forms the fruit?

Sol. Fruit is the seed-bearing structure in flowering plants formed from the ovary after flowering.

- *Apple is called a false fruit* because in an apple, the fleshy receptacle forms the main edible part. False fruits are those fruits which arise from other floral parts (like thalamus, receptacle, or calyx) except the ovary.
- *Ovary forms the fruit* after fertilisation or without fertilisation in parthenocarpic fruits.

Note

False fruits are also called as parthenocarpic fruits. Parthenocarpy is the phenomenon in which fruits are formed without fertilisation. Parthenocarpic fruits are seedless fruits. E.g. apple, pineapple, banana.

15. What is meant by emasculation? When and why does a plant breeder employ this technique?

Sol. • *Emasculation* is the removal of stamens (mainly the anthers) from the flower buds before their dehiscence. It does not affect the female reproductive part (pistil), which is used in various plant hybridisation techniques.

Emasculation *can be done in bisexual flowers* to obtain the desired variety of a plant by crossing a particular plant with the desired pollen grain. To remove the anthers, the flowers are covered with a bag before they open. This ensures that the flower is pollinated by pollen grains obtained from desirable varieties only. Later, the mature, viable, and stored pollen grains are dusted on the bagged stigma by breeders to allow artificial pollination to take place and obtain the desired plant variety.

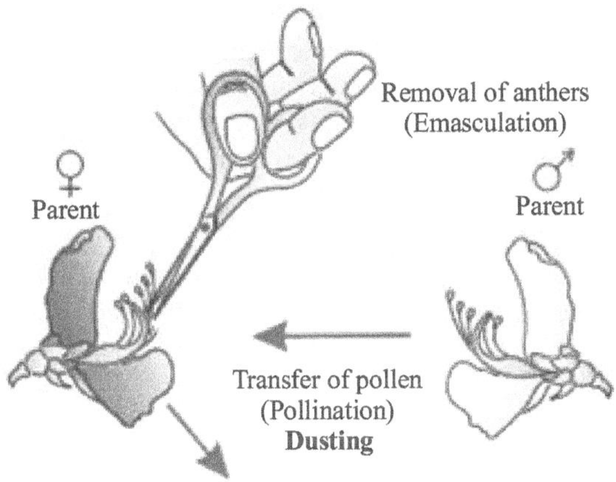

Fig.: Method of emasculation

- *Plant breeders employed this technique in artificial hybridisation,*
  - to prevent the pollination within same flower (self pollination).
  - to pollinate stigmas with pollens of desired variety to get disease-resistant plants and to avoid unwanted pollen rejection.

16. If one can induce parthenocarpy through the application of growth substances, which fruits would you select to induce parthenocarpy and why?

Sol. Parthenocarpic fruits are seedless fruits. They develop from ovary without fertilisation or seed formation. Such fruits can be induced by the application of plant growth hormones (such as auxin) to produce seedless fruit.

Therefore, the seedless varieties of economically important fruits such as oranges, pineapple, guava, watermelon, lemon, banana, grapes are selected to induce parthenocarpy.

17. Explain the role of tapetum in the formation of pollen-grain wall.

Sol. Tapetum is the innermost layer of the microsporangium. The tapetal cells are multinucleated and polyploid. It is located between sporangenous tissue and the anther wall. Tapetum is important for the nutrition and development of pollen grain, as well as a sources of precursors for the pollen coat.

- *Role of tapetum in the formation of pollen grain wall*
  During microsporogenesis, the cells of tapetum produce various enzymes, hormones, amino acids, and other nutritious material which are required for the development of pollen grains. Tapetal cells contain ubisch bodies that help in the ornamentation of the microspores or pollen grains walls (exine). The wall of the pollen grain consists of two layers: the inner intine wall and the outer exine wall. The inner layer, laid by the cells themselves consists, at least in part, of cellulose or hemicellulose. The outer layer of the pollen grain is called exine and is made up of the sporopollenin (secreted by the ubisch bodies of the tapetal cells). This compound provides spiny appearance to the exine of the pollen grains. The outer layer is the most durable layer and resistant to disintegration therefore treatment with intense heat, strong acids, or strong bases has very little effect upon it.

Note

Pollen grains are very common constituents of geologic sediments, both recent and ancient because of their high resistance to decay, their widespread dispersal by wind and water, and their abundant production by plants, Because of these features, pollen grains have provided much information on the origin and geologic history of terrestrial plant life.

18. What is apomixis and what is its importance?

Sol.

- *Apomixis* is a form of asexual reproduction that produces seeds without fertilisation, e.g., some species of asteraceae and grasses.
- *Importance of apomixis*
  (i) It helps in hybrid seed production. The method of producing hybrid seeds by cultivation is very expensive for farmers. Also, by sowing hybrid seeds, it is difficult to maintain hybrid characters as characters segregate during meiosis. This can be avoided if apomixis can be introduced in hybrid seeds.
  (ii) It prevents the loss of specific characters in the hybrid.
  (iii) It helps in producing hybrid varieties with increased yield.
  (iv) It is a cost-effective and time efficient method for producing seeds.

Note

Apomixis is a genetically controlled reproductive process whose major advantage over sexual reproduction is the possibility to select individuals with desirable gene combinations and to propagate them as clones. The ability to generate maternal clones and therefore rapidly fix desirable genotypes in crop species could accelerate agricultural breeding strategies.

Chapter 3

HUMAN REPRODUCTION

CHAPTER AT A GLANCE

- Human are **unisexual** and **viviparous**.
- Sexual reproduction is the only method of reproduction in humans.
- Reproductive structure in humans are divided into– male reproductive system and female reproductive system.
- The **major reproductive events in human beings** are:
  (i) Gametogenesis – Formation of gametes.
  (ii) Insemination – Transfer of sperms into female genital tract.
  (iii) Fertilisation – Fusion of male and female gametes leading to formation of zygote.
  (iv) Implantation – Formation and development of blastocyst and its attachment to the uterine wall.
  (v) Gestation – Time from conception to birth and embryonic development.
  (vi) Parturition – Delivery of baby (the process of birth).

  These reproductive events occur after puberty (= period when reproductive organs starts functioning).
- The characters which distinguish the male from the female externally are called **secondary sex characters**.

MALE REPRODUCTIVE SYSTEM

- Male reproductive system performs two major functions – spermatogenesis and transfer of sperm.
- It consists of a pair of testis, duct system & associated glands and external genitalia.
- **Testis** (the primary reproductive structure) are male gonads and produce male gametes (sperms) and male sex hormones (testosterone).
- Each testis has 250 compartments called testicular lobules. Each testicular lobules contain 1 – 3 seminiferous tubules.
- **Seminiferous tubule** is the site of sperm formation by a process called spermatogenesis. It is a place where germination, maturation, and transportation of the sperm cells take place.
- Seminiferous tubules are made up of columnar Sertoli cells surrounded by spermatogenic cells on the epithelial interior and stem cells exteriorly.
- The region outside the seminiferous tubule is called **interstitial space**. These spaces contain interstitial cells or Leydig cell.

- **Leydig cell** secretes male sex hormone (called testosterone) for the growth and maintenance of germinal epithelial cells and the development of secondary sex characteristics.
- Spermatogonia undergo meiosis and form sperms while sertoli cells (also called subtentacular cells) provide nutrition to the germs cells.
- **Male sex accessory ducts** include rete testis, vasa efferentia, epididymis, a vas deferens, and an ejaculatory duct. These ducts store and transport the sperms from the testis to the outside through **urethra**.
- **Vasa efferentia** carries spermatozoa from the rete testis to the epididymis.
- The **penis** is the male external genitalia. It contains urethra which serves as common canal for urine and semen.
- The **male accessory glands** include paired seminal vesicles, a prostate and paired bulbourethral glands.
- **Seminal vesicles** are the glands that contribute major portion of the seminal fluid.
- Secretions of seminal vesicle, prostate gland and bulbourethral gland are called **semen**.

FEMALE REPRODUCTIVE SYSTEM

- It consists of a pair of ovaries, oviducts, uterus, vagina and associated glands and external genitalia.
- **Ovaries** are female gonads and responsible for producing female sex hormones (oestrogen) and gametes (ova).
- Each ovary is covered by a thin epithelium which encloses the ovarian cortex.
- Scattered throughout the cortex are many rounded or oval bodies, called **ovarian or Graafian follicles** at various stages of development.
- Each follicle contains a large ovum surrounded by many layers of follicle cells.
- **Graafian follicle** is a mature ovarian follicle that contains a liquid-filled cavity (called antrum) and ruptures during ovulation to release an egg.
- Every month the most mature ovum from one ovary is released.
- At birth female ovaries contain 2 million follicles, each with an ovum that has begun meiosis but which is arrested in prophase of the first meiotic division. At this stage the ova are called primary oocyte.
- In the cortex both young and mature follicles along with a mass of yellow cells called **corpus luteum** is also present.
- Corpus luteum contain a yellow pigment lutein and secrete the hormone progesterone during pregnancy and hormone relaxin toward the end of pregnancy.
- **Oviducts (fallopian tubes)** is a pair of long duct which extends from the **periphery of each ovary to uterus**. It is the site of fertilisation.

- Fallopian tube is **divided into four parts: infundibulum** (a funnel-shaped opening near the ovary to which fimbriae are attached), **fimbriae** (finger-like, ciliated projections, responsible to capture the ovum from the surface of the ovary after ovulation), **ampulla** (widest section of the uterine tubes where fertilisation usually occurs) and **isthmus** (a narrow section of the uterine tubes connecting the ampulla to the uterine cavity).
- **Uterus (womb)** is a hollow muscular organ which receives embryo and provide optimal conditions for its survival and growth.
  It consists of three layers: **endometrium** (inner layer which is highly specialised and essential to menstrual and reproductive function), **myometrium** (middle layer which makes up most of the uterine volume and composed primarily of smooth muscle cells) and **perimetrium** (outer layer which is a thin layer of tissue made of epithelial cells that envelop the uterus).
- **Vagina** is meant to receive male's penis during copulation and also allow menstrual flow.
- **Bartholin's glands** secrete fluid which serves as a lubricant during copulation.
- **Mammary gland** is a gland located in the breasts of females that is responsible for lactation, or the production of milk. Mammary glands only produce milk after childbirth.
- The **basic components of the mammary gland** are the **alveoli** (hollow cavities, a few millimetres large) lined with milk-secreting cuboidal cells and surrounded by myoepithelial cells. These alveoli join up to form groups known as lobules, and each lobule has a lactiferous duct that drains into openings in the nipple.

GAMETOGENESIS

- **Gametogenesis** is a process in which a haploid sex cell (n) - sperm and ova are formed from a diploid primary germ cells (called gametogonia) present in the reproductive organs (called gonads-testes and ovary) through meiosis and cell differentiation.
- **Spermatogenesis**
  - Production of mature sperm cell in the testis is known as **spermatogenesis.** It starts at the age of puberty.
  - Spermatogonia (2N) divide mitotically into primary spermatocytes (2N), which divide by meiosis-I into secondary spermatocytes (1N).
  - Secondary spermatocytes (1N) transformed into spermatozoa (1N) by **spermiogenesis**.
  - Each spermatozoan or sperm is a long, flagellated, motile cell and consists of a **head** (comprising nucleus and acrosome), a **neck** (containing two centrioles), a **middle piece** (containing mitochondria) and a **tail**.

- **Oogenesis**
  - **Oogenesis** is the process of formation of mature female gamete called ova.
  - It is initiated during embryonic development stage when a couple of million gamete mother cell (oogonia) are formed within each foetal ovary.
  - When more layers of granulosa cell and a new theca are laid down then it is called **secondary follicles.**
  - The secondary follicle transform into a tertiary follicle which is characterised by a fluid filled cavity (called **antrum**).
  - Tertiary follicle further undergo changes into mature follicle (or **Graafian follicle**).
  - The Graafian follicle now ruptures to release the secondary oocyte from the ovary by a process called **ovulation.**
  - The **mature ovum or egg or secondary oocyte** is spherical in shape, contains nucleus & the **largest cell in the body**.
- If the secondary oocyte is fertilised by a sperm, chemical changes will trigger the completion of meiosis II and the formation of another polar body (the first polar body may also undergo a second division to form a third polar body).
- Once meiosis II is complete the mature egg forms an ovum, before fusing its nucleus with the sperm nucleus to form a zygote.
- Ovum is larger and non- motile without the flagella.

MENSTRUAL CYCLE

- It involves cyclic changes in female's reproductive tract culminating in menstruation that is flow of cast off uterine and fallopian tube lining along with blood and tissue fluid through the vagina.
- Beginning of menstruation or first menstruation at puberty (called **menarche**) usually varies. It usually occurs between 12 and 15 years.
- When menstrual cycles permanently cease due to the natural depletion of ovarian oocytes from aging, the condition is called **menopause.**
- Menopause marks the permanent end of fertility and the average age of menopause is 51 years.
- Two **key groups of hormones which control and coordinate the menstrual cycle** are pituitary and ovarian hormones.

  Pituitary hormones (FSH and LH) are released from the anterior pituitary gland and act on the ovaries to develop follicles. Ovarian hormones (oestrogen and progesterone) are released from the ovaries and act on the uterus to prepare for pregnancy.
- Menstrual cycle consists of **menstrual phase, proliferative phase** (follicular phase) and **secretory phase** (luteal phase).

FERTILISATION AND EMBRYONIC DEVELOPMENT

- During copulation, the semen is transferred into the vagina. The motile sperms and the ovum released from the ovary reaches the ampullary-isthmic junction, where fertilisation takes place.

- **Fertilisation** is a process in which male and female gametes are fused together, initiating the development of a new organism with the combination of genes of both the parents. The product of fertilisation is a cell called **zygote**.
- After the formation of zygote, it starts moving through fallopian tube towards the uterus.
- The zygote undergoes successive (mitotic) divisions called **cleavage** (also called segmentation), as it moves through the isthmus of fallopian tube towards the uterus and form **blastocyst** which embedded in the endometrium; this process is called **implantation** and its leads to pregnancy.
- After implantation chorionic villi & uterine tissue interdigitated with each other & jointly form a structural & functional unit between developing embryo & maternal body called **placenta**.
- Placenta supply oxygen & nutrients to the embryo & remove carbon dioxide & excretory/waste materials produced by the embryo.
- Expulsion of the young one at the end of gestation is known as **parturition**. Parturition is induced by a complex neuro-endocine mechanism. The signals for parturition originate from the fully developed foetus and the placenta which induce mild uterine contraction called **foetal-ejection reflex**.
- Gestation period is **280 days in humans**.

LACTATION

- **Lactation** is a process of milk production. Human milk is secreted by the mammary glands, which are located within the fatty tissue of the breast.
- The natural production of breast milk (lactation) is triggered by a complex interaction between three hormones -oestrogen, progesterone and human placental lactogen - during the final months of pregnancy.
- The mammary glands undergo differentiation during pregnancy and starts producing milk towards the end of pregnancy.
- The milk produced during the initial few days of lactation is called **colostrum**.
- Colostrum is especially high in nutrients, fats, and antibodies, to protect the newborn from infection.

EXERCISE

1. **Fill in the blanks:**
   (a) **Humans reproduce ______(asexually/sexually).**
   (b) **Humans are ______ (oviparous, viviparous, ovoviviparous).**
   (c) **Fertilisation is ______ in humans (external/internal).**
   (d) **Male and female gametes are ______ (diploid/haploid).**
   (e) **Zygote is ______ (diploid/haploid).**
   (f) **The process of release of ovum from a mature follicle is called ______.**
   (g) **Ovulation is induced by a hormone called ______.**
   (h) **The fusion of male and female gametes is called ______.**
   (i) **Fertilisation takes place in ______.**
   (j) **Zygote divides to form ______which is implanted in uterus.**
   (k) **The structure which provides vascular connection between foetus and uterus is called ______.**

Sol. (a) sexually (b) viviparous
(c) internal (d) haploid
(e) diploid (f) ovulation
(g) LH (luteinising hormone)
(h) fertilisation
(i) ampullary-isthmic junction (fallopian tube)
(j) blastocyst
(k) placenta (umbilical cord)

2. Draw a labelled diagram of male reproductive system.

Sol. Male reproductive system produces, maintain, and transport sperm (the male reproductive cells) and protective fluid (semen) within the female reproductive tract during sex.

Labelled diagram of male reproductive system is given below:

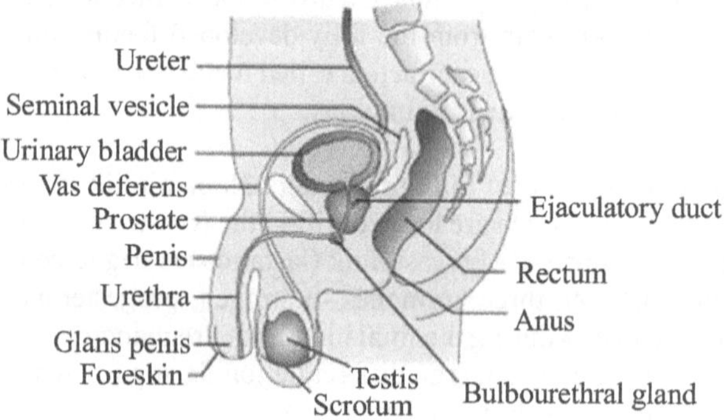

(a)

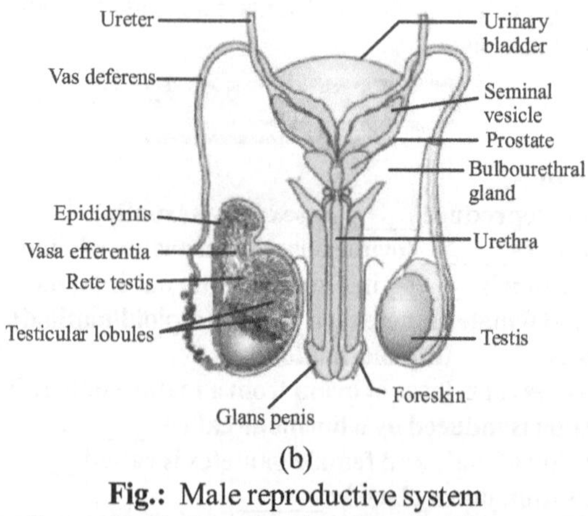

(b)

Fig.: Male reproductive system
(a) Diagrammatic sectional view of male pelvis showing reproductive system
(b) Diagrammatic view of male reproductive system

3. Draw a labelled diagram of female reproductive system.

Sol. Female reproductive system produces eggs, sex hormones like oestrogen, progesterone and maintains reproduction and pregnancy.

Labelled diagram of female reproductive system is given below:

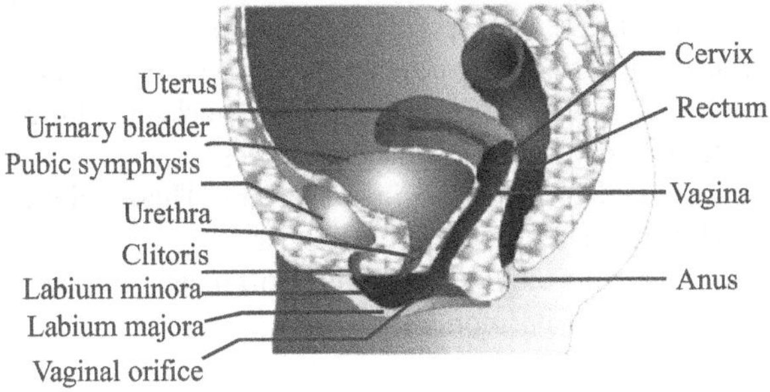

(a)

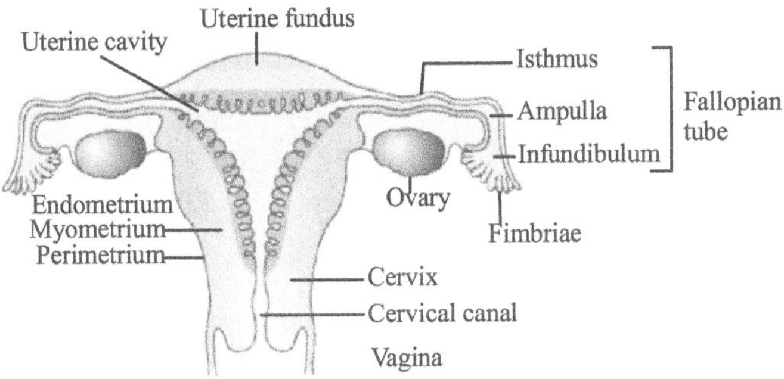

(b)

Fig.: Female reproductive system

(a) Diagrammatic sectional view of female pelvis showing reproductive system

(b) Diagrammatic sectional view of the female reproductive system

4. Write two major functions each of testis and ovary.

Sol.
- **Testes** – Testes are the primary sexual organs in male. Two *major functions* of testes are :
  (i) Testosterone production from Leydig cells of seminiferous tubule.
  (ii) Production of sperm cells in seminiferous tubules through spermatogenesis.
- **Ovary** – Ovaries are the primary female sex organs. Two *main functions* of ovaries are :
  (i) Productions of female germ cells called eggs or oocytes through oogenesis.
  (ii) Production of hormones – oestrogens & progesterone which affect many of the female secondary sexual characters & reproductive functions.

5. Describe the structure of a seminiferous tubule.

Sol. Seminiferous tubule is a structural unit located within the testis. These tubules are enclosed by a thick basal lamina and surrounded by 3-4 layers of smooth muscle cells (or myoid cells). The insides of the tubules are lined with seminiferous epithelium, which consists of two general types of cells: Sertoli or supporting cells & spermatogenic cells.

Sertoli cells, are elongated and pyramidal & partially envelop the spermatogenic cells. Sertoli cells have pale nuclei and dense nucleoli. These cells provide nourishment to the developing spermatogenic cells.

Spermatogenic cells are stacked in 4-8 layers. These cells divide several times & differentiate to produce spermatozoa.

Between seminiferous tubules lie the interstitial cells or Leydig cells which produces testosterone hormone.

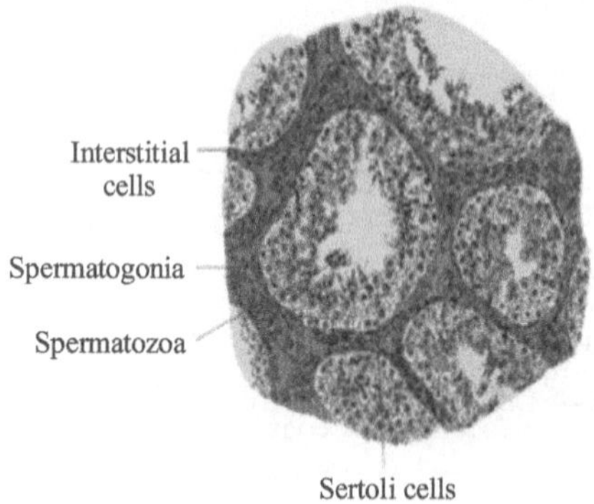

Fig.: Structure of seminiferous tubule

The seminiferous tubules function to produce sperm, maintain sperm, and store the sperm. During the process of meiosis the Sertoli cells that line the seminiferous tubules undergo the process of differentiation to be converted into sperm.

6. What is spermatogenesis? Briefly describe the process of spermatogenesis.

Sol.
- *Spermatogenesis* is the process of producing sperms from primordial germ cells with half the number of chromosomes (haploid) as somatic cells. It takes place in seminiferous tubules.
- *Process of spermatogenesis* : Sperm production begins at puberty continues throughout life with several hundred million sperms being produced each day. Once sperm are formed they move into the epididymis, where they mature and are stored.

  Spermatogenesis starts due to significant increase in the secretion of gonadotropin releasing hormone (GnRH) from hypothalamus.

  During spermatogenesis one spermatogonium produces 4 sperms.

  Spermatogenesis completes through the following phases – multiplicative phase, growth phase, maturation phase & spermiogenesis.

(i) In *multiplicative phase*, the sperm mother cells divide by mitosis & produce spermatogonia.

(ii) The spermatogonia grow in size to form large primary spermatocytes by getting nourishment from sertoli cells in *growth phase.*

(iii) *Maturation phase* involves meiosis I in which primary spermatocytes divide to produce secondary spermatocyte and meiosis II which produces spermatids. Thus, each primary spermatocyte gives rise to four haploid spermatids.

(iv) *Spermiogenesis or spermateliosis* is process of formation of flagellated spermatozoa from spermatids. Spermiogenesis begins in the seminiferous tubules but usually completed in epididymis. During spermiogenesis, the acrosome forms, the flagellar apparatus forms, and most excess cytoplasm (the residual body) is separated and left in the Sertoli cell. Spermatozoa are released into the lumen of the seminiferous tubule. A small amount of excess cytoplasm (the cytoplasmic droplet) is shed later in the epididymis.

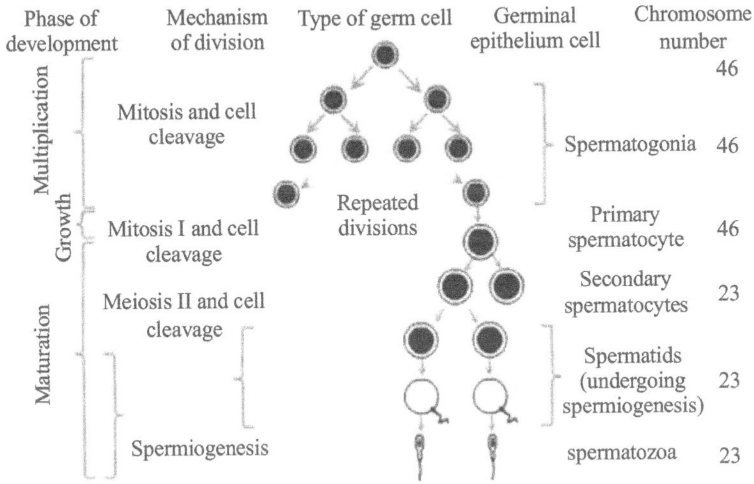

Fig.: Spermatogenesis

7. Name the hormones involved in regulation of spermatogenesis.

Sol. *Hormones involved in the regulation of spermatogenesis* are GnRH, LH, FSH and inhibin.

After sexual maturity, spermatogenesis starts due to the secretion of gonadotropin releasing hormone (GnRH) from the hypothalamus of brain.

GnRH acts on pituitary gland and stimulates secretion of luteinising hormone (LH) and follicle stimulating hormone (FSH).

A negative feedback system occurs in the male with rising levels of testosterone acting on the hypothalamus and anterior pituitary to inhibit the release of GnRH, FSH, and LH.

The Sertoli cells produce the hormone inhibin, which is released into the blood when the sperm count is too high.

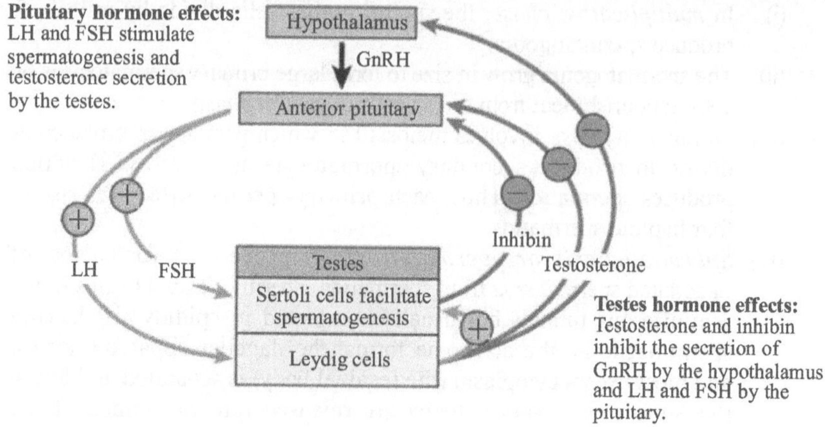

Fig.: Regulation of spermatogenesis

8. Define spermiogenesis and spermiation.

Sol.
- *Spermiogenesis* is the process of transformation of spermatids into mature flagellated spermatozoa (sperms).
- *Spermiation* is the process of release of mature spermatozoa from the sertoli cells. In this spermatozoa are shed into the lumen of seminiferous tubule for transport.

9. Draw a labelled diagram of sperm.

Sol. Sperm are the only human cells that contain flagella. They are made up of three basic parts- head, middle piece and tail.

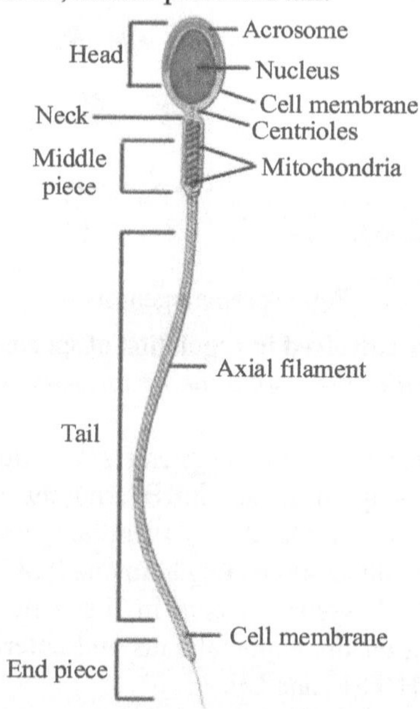

Fig.: Sperm

10. What are the major components of seminal plasma?

Sol. Semen, also called seminal fluid (produced in male), is composed of sperms and seminal plasma. Seminal plasma is the fluid in which sperm is ejaculated. *Major components of seminal plasma* are secretions from seminal vesicles, prostrate and bulbourethral gland; sperms from testis and mucus.

Seminal plasma is rich in fructose and contains enzymes, citric acid, hormones like prostaglandins, calcium and clotting proteins. It provides nourishment and protection to sperms.

Note

Seminal vesicles are major contributors to the production of semen.

11. What are the major functions of male accessory ducts and glands?

Sol.
- The male accessory ducts are vasa efferentia, epididymis, vas deferens, and rete testis. *Major functions of male accessory ducts* are as follows:
  - It aid in sperm transport.
  - It acts as a temporary storage of spermatozoa.
- Male accessory glands in humans are the seminal vesicles, prostate gland, and the bulbourethral glands (also called Cowper's glands). The *major function of these glands* is to secrete fluids that enter the urethra. Secretions of these glands constitute the seminal plasma which are rich in fructose, ascorbic acid, citrate, calcium, certain enzymes and prostaglandins. These secretions lubricates the reproductive system and nourish and activate the spermatozoa to swim.

12. What is oogenesis? Give a brief account of oogenesis.

Sol.
- The process of formation of a mature female gamete (ovum) is called *oogenesis*. It occurs in the ovaries of female reproductive system. It is a discontinuous process as it begins before birth, stops in midprocess & only resumes after menarch.
- *Process of oogenesis* : It occurs in three phases :

  (i) *Multiplicative phase*: The initial phase of oogenesis starts during foetal stage. The primordial germinal cells divide repeatedly to form the oogonia. The oogonia are known to divide again several times mitotically to produce a large number of cells called the primary oocytes. After the formation of primary oocytes there is no more division. The cells enter into the growth phase.

  (ii) *Growth phase*: In the growth phase, the size of the primary oocyte increases enormously.

  (iii) *Maturation phase*: During this phase, diploid primary oocyte transformed into mature through meiosis.

Maturation phase produces two haploid cells – Larger one called secondary oocyte & the smaller one called polar bodies (1st polar body). Meiosis II of secondary oocyte results in the formation of functional egg or ovum and a second polar body. The first polar body may also divide to form two polar bodies of equal sizes which do not take part in reproduction & ultimately degenerates. First maturation division may be completed in the ovaries just prior to ovulation but second one (final) is completed outside the ovary after fertilisation. The egg is released at secondary oocyte stage under the effect of LH.

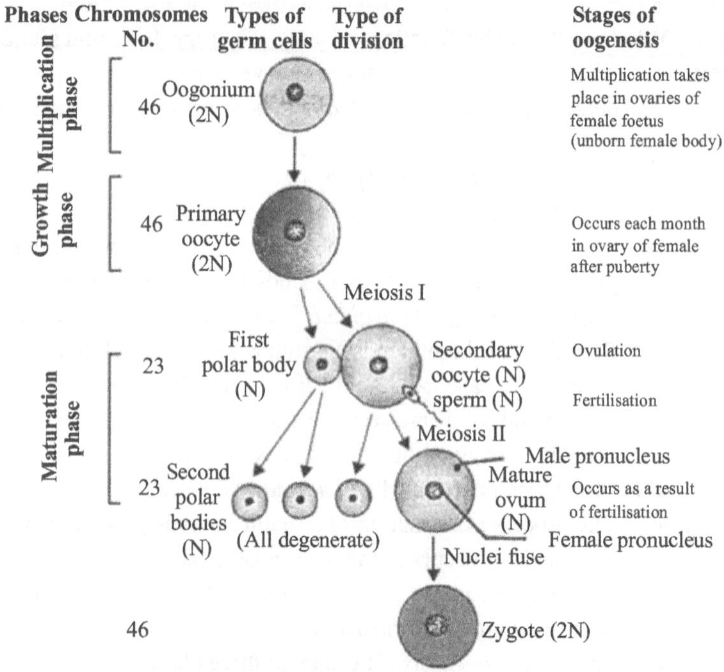

Fig.: Oogenesis

> **Note**
>
> - *The growth phase of oogenesis is longer and more complicated than in spermatogenesis.*
> - *The primary oocyte completes its first meiotic division producing a secondary oocyte and the first polar body. The secondary oocyte enters meiosis II and is arrested at metaphase II.*

13. Draw a Labelled diagram of a section through ovary.

Sol. Ovary is an female reproductive organ that produces an ovum and female sex hormones (like oestrogen).

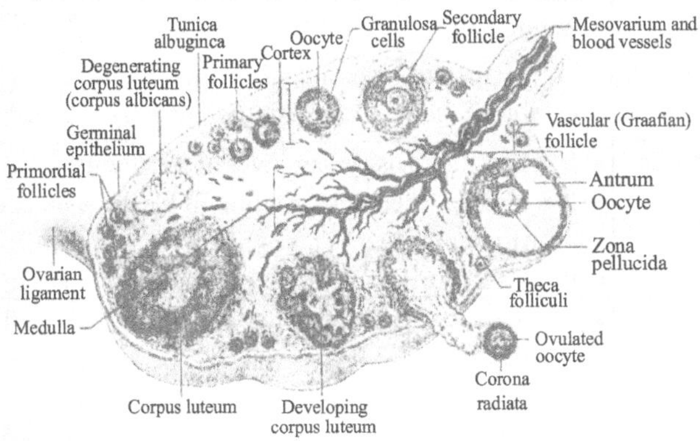

Fig.: Labelled diagram of ovary

14. Draw a labelled diagram of a Graafian follicle.

Sol. Graafian follicle is a mature fluid filled cavity in the ovary that ruptures during ovulation to release an egg (secondary oocyte).

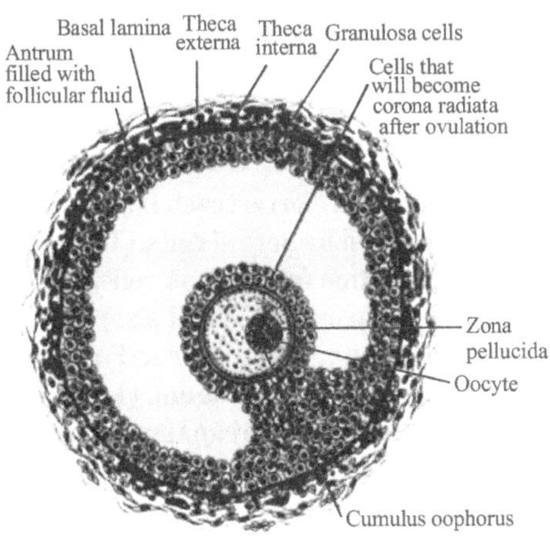

Fig.: Graafian follicle

15. Name the functions of the following:

(a) Corpus luteum

(b) Endometrium

(c) Acrosome

(d) Sperm tail

(e) Fimbriae

Sol.

	Term	Function
(a)	Corpus luteum	• It is a temporary endocrine organ that plays an integral role in regulation of the menstrual cycle and early pregnancy. • It secretes progesterone hormone which is essential for establishing and maintaining pregnancy in females.
(b)	Endometrium	• It is the innermost lining layer of the uterus. • It is a place where implantation of blastocysts and formation of placenta takes place. • It is also involved in the development of embryo.
(c)	Acrosome	• It develops over the anterior half of the head in the spermatozoa. • It help the sperm get through the egg's protective coat with the help of hydrolytic enzymes released during acrosome reaction. • It allows the plasma membranes of the sperm and egg to fuse during fertilisation.
(d)	Sperm tail	• It helps in propelling or swim the sperm cell forward to meet the egg.
(e)	Fimbriae	• It is responsible for capturing the egg when it is released from the ovary. • It also help egg to move from the ovaries to uterus.

16. Identify True/False statements. Correct each false statement to make it true.

(a) Androgens are produced by Sertoli cells. (True/False)

(b) Spermatozoa get nutrition from sertoli cells. (True/False)

(c) Leydig cells are found in ovary. (True/False)

(d) Leydig cells synthesise androgens. (True/False)

(e) Oogenesis takes place in corpus luteum. (True/False)

(f) Menstrual cycle ceases during pregnancy. (True/False)

(g) Presence or absence of hymen is not a reliable indicator of virginity or sexual experience. (True/False)

Sol. (a) *False*. Androgens or male sex hormones (e.g. testosterone) are secreted by Leydig cells found in the seminiferous tubule of the testis.

(b) *True*. Sertoli cells are the somatic cells of the testis that are essential for testis formation and spermatogenesis. Its main function is to nourish the developing sperm cells through the stages of spermatogenesis, hence, also been called the "mother" or "nurse" cell. Sertoli cells also act as phagocytes, consuming the residual cytoplasm during spermatogenesis.

(c) *False*. Leydig cells are found in testis.

(d) *True*. Leydig cells, also known as interstitial cells of Leydig produce testosterone (androgen) in the presence of luteinising hormone (LH).

(e) *False.* Oogenesis takes place in ovary and lead to formation of a single egg cell or ovum.

(f) *True.* Menstrual cycle ceases during pregnancy because if the woman gets pregnant around the mid-cycle, the foetus's placenta starts secreting Human Chorionic Gonadotropin (HCG). HCG causes the remnant of the ruptured follicle to start growing (and make the yellow body, corpus luteum) and start secreting progesterone for maintaining the pregnancy.

(g) *True.* Presence or absence of the hymen is not a reliable indicator of virginity or sexual experience because hymen is a very thin membrane which exists at the opening of the vagina and it can easily be broken due to following reasons: during the first coitus (intercourse), sudden fall or jolt, insertion of a vaginal tampon, active participation in some sports like horseback riding, cycling, etc.

17. What is menstrual cycle? Which hormones regulate menstrual cycle?

Sol.
- *Menstrual cycle* is the cyclic change in the reproductive tract of primate female. This period is marked by a characteristic event repeated almost every month (28 days with minor variation) in the form of a menstrual flow (*i.e.* shedding of the endometrium of the uterus with bleeding). It may be temporarily stopped only in pregnancy.
- The *hormones that regulates menstrual cycles* are:
  - FSH (Follicle stimulating hormone) and LH (Luteinising hormone) (secreted from anterior pitutary gland)
  - Oestrogen (secreted from ovary)
  - Progesterone (secreted from corpus luteum).

18. What is parturition? Which hormones are involved in induction of parturition?

Sol.
- Vigorous contraction of the uterus at the end of pregnancy causes expulsion/delivery of the foetus. This process of delivery of the foetus is called *parturition (child birth).*
- Parturition is *induced by hormone oxytocin* which acts on the uterine muscle and causes stronger uterine contractions.

19. In our society the women are often blamed for giving birth to daughters. Can you explain why this is not correct?

Sol. All human beings contain 23 pairs of chromosomes in which 22 pair of chromosomes are autosomes and one pair of sex chromosome.

The sex chromosome pattern in the human females is XX and that of male is XY. Therefore, all the haploid female gametes (ova) have the sex chromosome X, however, the haploid male gametes have either X or Y. Thus 50% of sperms carry the X-chromosome while the other 50% carry the Y-chromosome. After fusion of the male and female gametes, the zygote carries either XX or XY depending upon whether the sperm carrying X or Y fertilizes the ovum. The zygote carrying XX would be a female baby and XY would be a male baby. That is why it is correct to say that the sex of the baby is determined by the father.

20. How many eggs are released by a human ovary in a month? How many eggs do you think would have been released if the mother gave birth to identical twins? Would your answer change if the twins born were fraternal?

Sol.
- *One egg is released* by human ovary in a month.
- *Identical twins* : Identical twins are formed when a single fertilised egg splits into two genetically identical parts. The twins share the same DNA set, thus they may share many similar attributes. However, since physical appearance is influenced by environmental factors and not just genetics, identical twins can actually look very different.
- *Fraternal twins* : These twins are formed when two fertilised eggs are formed. The twins share the different DNA set, thus they may share different attributes (dizygotic embryo).

21. How many eggs do you think were released by the ovary of a female dog which gave birth to 6 puppies?

Sol. Dogs and rodents are polyovulatory species. In these species, more than one ovum is released from the ovary at the time of ovulation. Hence, *six eggs are released by the ovary of a female dog to produce six puppies*.

Chapter

4 REPRODUCTIVE HEALTH

CHAPTER AT A GLANCE

- **Reproductive health** refers to as a total well being in physical, emotional, behavioural and social aspects of reproduction at all stages of life.
- Health is affected by: genetic disorders and deficiencies with which an individual is born; infections and life style that includes - food and water, rest, exercise and habits.
- India was the first in the world to initiate various action plans/programmes at national level to attain total reproductive health as a social goal.
- The rapid increase in human population size over a relatively short period is called **human population explosion**.
- **Causes of population explosion**
  - Reduced death rate
  - Increased food production
  - Improvement of public health and medical facility
  - Increase in number of people in reproductive age.
  - Decreased infant motility rate (IMR) and maternal mortality rate (MMR).
- Overpopulation has resulted in serious problems like depletion of natural resources, various socio-economic problems, energy crisis and ecodegradation.
  - Socio-economic problems are shortage of food supply, space, unemployment, essential goods and poverty
  - Energy crisis – Increase in population has created greater demand for energy – fuel wood, fossil fuel etc.
  - Ecodegradation are pollution and sanitation.

BIRTH CONTROL

- The birth control methods which deliberately prevent pregnancy by interfering with normal process of ovulation, fertilisation and implantation are referred to as **contraception**.
- **Contraceptive methods** are preventive methods to help woman avoid unwanted pregnancies. These methods are of two types – temporary & permanent.
- **Temporary methods** include natural methods and barriers method.
- **Natural methods** prevents the chances of sperm with ovum meeting. It can be acquired by safe period, coitus interruptus, abstinence, lactational amenorrhea.
  - **Safe period :** A weak before & a week after the menses is considered as the safe period (rhythm method) for sexual intercourse.
  - **Coitus interruptus** involves the withdrawal of the penis by the male before the ejaculation so that semen is not deposited in the vagina & there is no fertilisation.

- **Abstinence** is a way to avoid conception by abstain from sexual intercourse.
- **Lactational amenorrhea** (absence of menstruation) method is based on the fact that ovulation & therefore the cycle do not occur during the period of intense lactation following parturition. It is a temporary postnetal infertility.

- **Barrier methods** utilises a block or boundary, to keep sperm from penetrating the egg. It includes spermicides, condoms, diaphragms, cervical cap, intrauterine devices (IUDs) etc.
  - **Spermicidal creams, jellies** and **foams** are chemical barriers. They are usually used along with these barriers to increase their contraceptive efficiency. They prevent conception by blocking the entry of sperms into the female body. These devices are **reusable.**
  - **Condom** (Nirodh), a type of mechanical barrier, is a rubber sheath to cover the erect penis in male and vagina and cervix in females just before the coitus to avoid the insemination. This helps in preventing the conception by blocking meeting of sperm and ova. It is also a safeguard against AIDS & other sexual diseases.
  - **Diaphragms & cervical cap** are rubber plastic covers that are fitted on the cervix & check the entry of sperms into the uterus.
  - **Intrauterine devices (IUDs)** are plastic or metal devices placed in the uterus. They contain either copper or a common synthetic hormone used in oral contraceptives. These include loop, copper-T, spiral etc. They prevent fertilisation of the egg or implantation of egg.
- **Oral contraceptives (birth control pills)** check ovulation by inhibiting the secretion of FSH & LH hormone that are necessary for ovulation.
- Most birth control pill contain small doses of either progesterone or progesterone-oestrogen combinations. Pills have to be taken daily for a period of 21 days starting preferably within the first five days of menstrual cycle.
- **Contraceptive implant** is made up of small thin flexible rod. They can be used under the skin. It consists of progesterone alone or in combination with oestrogen. Their action is similar to that of pills. It releases small amount of progestogen which stop ovulation and thicken the mucus in cervix (the entrance to uterus), making it difficult for sperm to get through and fertilise an egg.
- **Permanent methods** includes vasectomy in male and tubectomy in female.
  - **Vasectomy** in male involves a cut in the scrotal sac, cutting or burning of the vas deferens (tubes that carry sperm) & blocking both the cut ends. Vasectomy prevents the passage of sperm into seminal fluid.
  - Female sterilisation (called **tubectomy**) prevents fertilisation by interrupting the passage through fallopian tube. Eggs continues to be produced but they fail to pass into the uterus.
- **Medical termination of pregnancy** (MTPs) or induced abortion is one of the most widely used methods of fertility control in the world.

- MTP's are considered relatively safe during the first trimester *i.e.* upto 12 weeks of pregnancy.
- **Amniocentesis** is a prenatal diagnostic technique in which a sample of amniotic fluid from the womb of a pregnant woman is taken during the early stages of foetal development and the cells are cultured and analysed.
  By this method the chromosomal abnormalities, the sex of the foetus and development disorders could be detected. It is misused for female foeticides.
- **Sexually transmitted diseases (STDs)** are the diseases or infections which are transmitted through sexual intercourse with infected persons.
- Common STDs includes AIDS, gonorrhoea, syphilis, genital herpes, hepatitis-B etc.
  AIDS, genital herpes and hepatitis B cannot be cured while the others are curable STDs if detected early and treated properly.

INFERTILITY

- A large number of couples are infertile, *i.e.,* they are unable to produce children inspite of unprotected intercourse. Hence, infertility may be defined as the inability of a sexually active, non-contracepting couple to achieve pregnancy in one or two years.
- In cases where in corrective treatment of infertility is not possible, couples are assisted to have children through special programmes called **Assisted Reproduction Technologies** (ART).
- ART programme includes :
  (i) Test tube baby programme
  (ii) Gamete intrafallopian transfer (GIFT)
  (iii) Intra-cytoplasmic sperm injection (ICSI)
  (iv) Artificial insemination technique
- **Test Tube Baby Programme :** In this programme the fusion of ovum and sperm is done outside the body of woman to form a zygote which is allowed to divide to form embryo. This embryo is then implanted in uterus where it develops into a foetus which in turn develops into a child. This is called test tube baby. In this method, ova from the wife or a donor female and the sperms from the husband or a donor are allowed to fuse under simulated conditions (as that of the body) *in vitro* fertilisation.
- **Gamete Intra Fallopian Transfer (GIFT) :** This method involves the transfer of an ovum collected from a donor female into another female, who cannot produce ova, but can provide suitable conditions for fertilisation and further development of the foetus upto parturition.
- **Intra Cytoplasmic Sperm Injection (ICSI) :** In this method, the sperm is directly injected into the ovum to form an embryo in the laboratory and then embryo transfer is carried out.
- **Artificial insemination :** In this method, the semen collected from the husband or a healthy donor, is artificially introduced into the vagina or into the uterus (intra-uterine insemination) around the time of ovulation.

EXERCISE

1. What do you think is the significance of reproductive health in a society?

Sol. Reproductive health refers to the diseases, disorders and conditions that affects the functioning of the male and female reproductive systems during all stages of life.

Reproductive health in a society is significant because the people are aware of the following:

(i) Birth control methods and advantages of small family.

(ii) Sexually transmitted diseases like AIDS, syphilis etc. and methods to avoid them.

(iii) Importance of breast feeding and post-natal care of the mother and baby.

(iv) Equal opportunities for the male and female children.

(v) Sex abuse and sex related crimes etc.

(vi) Better sex education and awareness which helps to maintain the population and prevent population explosion.

(vii) Better family planning which lead to reduction of family size.

> **Note**
>
> *Spreading awareness regarding uncontrolled population growth and social evils among youth individual's will help in building up a reproductive healthy society.*

2. Suggest the aspects of reproductive health which need to be given special attention in the present scenario.

Sol. Reproductive health deals with the reproductive processes, functions and system at all stages of life.

The *aspects of reproductive health* which need to be given special attention in the present scenario are as follows:

(i) Creating awareness among the people regarding various reproductive-related aspects. It can be done through Government and non-government agencies, giving sex-education in the schools, parents and other relatives, teachers etc.

(ii) Creating awareness on providing and improving existing medical facilities and attention to the problems like menstrual irregularities, pregnancy related aspects, delivery, medical termination of pregnancy, STDs, birth control, infertility.

(iii) Post-natal child maternal management is another important aspect of the reproductive and child health care programme.

3. Is sex education necessary in schools? Why?

Sol.
- Yes, sex education is necessary in school.
- Introducing *sex education in the schools* of India is an *important issue because of the following reasons*:

(i) It encourage to provide the right or correct information to the young peoples so as to discourage children from believing in myths & having misconceptions about sex related aspects.
(ii) Proper information about reproductive organs, safe & hygienic sexual practices, STD's etc. would help people, those in the adolescent age group to lead a healthy reproductive life
(iii) Physical changes during adolescence are fully explained hence help can be provided if there is any abnormality. Changes in behaviour are predicted. It prevents development of mental problems.

In many countries, sexual education raises much contentious debate. Chief among the controversial points is whether covering **child sexuality** is valuable or detrimental; the use of birth control such as **condoms** and **hormonal contraception**, and the impact of such use on pregnancy, outside marriage, teenage pregnancy, and the transmission of STDs. Increasing support for abstinence – only sex education by conservative groups has been one of the primary causes of these controversies.

4. Do you think that reproductive health in our country has improved in the past 50 years? If yes, mention some such areas of improvement.

Sol.
- Yes, in the last 50 years, reproductive health in our country has improved.
- *Area of such improvement* is given below:
  (i) Massive child immunisation, which lead to decrease in child or infant mortality.
  (ii) Maternity and child health, due to better post-natal care of mother and baby.
  (iii) Increasing use of contraceptives, this result in a decrease in the rate of transmission of sexually transmitted diseases.
  (iv) Family planning, which create awareness of having small and healthy family.

  Bringing sexual and reproductive health services to the millions of people living in countries which still suffer from short life expectancies, high levels of child and maternal mortality, child labour and illiteracy and poor overall health remains a major challenge for governments and non government organisations.

5. What are the suggested reasons for population explosion?

Sol. Population explosion may be defined as a sudden and rapid rise on population growth. The *suggested reasons for population explosion* are:
(i) Increased health facilities along with better living conditions had an explosive impact on the growth of population.
(ii) Decline in death rate.
(iii) Decline in maternal mortality rate (MMR).
(iv) Decline in infant mortality rate (IMR).
(v) Increase in the number of people in the reproductive age.
(vi) Immigration to better developed countries due to several reasons like better job, opportunities, war and natural causes like hurricanes, earthquakes and so on.

6. Is the use of contraceptives justified? Give reasons.

Sol. A contraceptive is a device or drug that prevents a woman from becoming pregnant. It helps to protect against both sexually transmitted infections (STIs) and pregnancy.

Yes, the use of contraceptives is justified due to the following reasons:

(i) To overcome the population growth rate, contraceptive methods are used.

(ii) It will help in bringing birth rate down & subsequently curb population growth.

(iii) With the rapid spread of HIV/AIDS in the country, there is now a growing realisation about the need to know about contraceptions & condoms.

(iv) They are also helpful in preventing unwanted pregnancies.

(v) They do not interfere with sexual desire of sexual act.

7. Removal of gonads cannot be considered as a contraceptive option. Why?

Sol. Gonads are male and female primary reproductive gland that produces reproductive cells (called gametes-sperm and egg) for reproduction and secrete sex hormones which are needed for the growth and development of primary and secondary reproductive organs and structures. In males the gonads are called testes whereas in females they are called ovaries.

Removal of gonads or its parts *cannot be considered as a contraceptive option* because they are not used to prevent unwanted pregnancies and spreading of STDs . Removal of gonads are usually referred to as surgical methods of sterilisation which will lead to permanent infertility and also it will stop the secretions of essential sex hormones that are required for the normal functioning of the accessory reproductive parts.

Two important methods of sterilisation are called vasectomy and tubectomy which are carried out respectively in males and females. In both the condition, & both male and female will be dependent on hormones in their remaining life to regulate functioning of reproductive organs. These are very effective but their irreversibility is very poor, hence they are not considered as a good options for contraception.

8. Amniocentesis for sex determination is banned in our country. Is this ban necessary? Comment.

Sol. *Yes*, the *statutory ban on amniocentesis in our country is necessary*, because it is misused to find out the sex of the foetus leading to female foeticides.

Amniocentesis is the prenatal diagnostic technique, that helps to find out chromosomal (genetic) disorders, metabolic disorders of the foetus. It is carried out in the early second trimester of pregnancy. In this procedure amniotic fluid is removed that surrounds and protects the baby during pregnancy. The fluid contain foetal cells and various chemicals produced by the baby.

The solution to the problem is not passing more laws, such as banning sex determination ultrasounds but raising the social & economic status of women.

9. Suggest some methods to assist infertile couples to have children.

Sol.
- Infertility is the inability of a sexually active, non-contracepting couple to achieve pregnancy in one year. Specialised health care units (infertility clinics) could help in diagnosis and corrective treatment of some of these disorders and enable these couples to have children. However, where such corrections are not possible, the infertile couples could be assisted to have children through certain special techniques commonly known as ART (Assisted Reproductive Technologies).
  Success rates vary depending on many factors like age of the partners, reason for infertility, type of ART, if the egg is fresh or frozen.
- *Various methods of ART available* to help such couples are as follows:
  (i) *In vitro* fertilisation (IVF): It is a process in which egg is fertilised by sperm in a test tube or elsewhere outside the body. It is commonly known as the 'Test tube baby' programme. In this procedure eggs (ova) from a woman's ovary are removed and are fertilised with sperm in a laboratory procedure, and then the fertilized egg (embryo) is transferred to the woman's uterus for further development. The babies produced from this method are known as test tube babies.
  (ii) *Zygote Intra Fallopian Transfer (ZIFT)*: ZIFT is used when blockage in the fallopian tubes prevents the normal binding of sperm to the egg. In this procedure, egg is fertilised *in vitro* (outside the body) and then the zygote or early embryos (up to 8 blastomeres) is transferred into the fallopian tube.
  (iii) *Intra Uterine Transfer (IUT)*: Embryos with more than 8 blastomeres could be transferred into the uterus, to complete its further development. Embryos formed by *in vivo* fertilisation (fusion of gametes within the female) also could be used for such transfer to assist those females who cannot conceive.
  (iv) *Gamete Intra Fallopian Transfer (GIFT)*: In this technique, eggs are retrieved from a woman, mixed with sperm & immediately transferred to recipient female's fallopian tube that are unable to produce eggs but has the ability to conceive.
  (v) *Artificial insemination (AI)* : In this technique, the semen is collected either from husband or a healthy donor & is artificially introduced either into the vagina or into the uterus of the female (IUI-Intra uterine insemination). It is employed when the male partner is not able to inseminate the female or have low sperm count.
  (vi) *Intra Cytoplasmic Sperm Injection (ICSI)* : In this method, sperm & eggs are retrieved from both the parents. A single sperm is injected directly into an egg, and then the fertilised egg is implanted into the woman's uterus.

10. What are the measures one has to take to prevent from contracting STDs?

Sol. Sexually transmitted diseases (STDs) get transferred from one individual to the other through sexual contact. Adolescents and young adults are at the greatest risk of acquiring these sexually transmitted diseases.

STDs can be prevented by the following measures:

(i) Use sterile needles if injecting intravenous drugs.

(ii) Delay having sexual relationships as long as possible. The younger a person is when he or she begins to have sex for the first time, the more susceptible he or she becomes to developing an STD.

(iii) Learn the symptoms of STDs and seek medical help as soon as possible if any symptoms develop.

(iv) Avoid having sexual intercourse during menstruation.

(v) Avoid sex with unknown partner/multiple partners.

(vi) Always use condoms during intercourse.

(vii) In case of doubt, go for medical professional for early detection and get complete treatment if diagnosed with disease.

(viii) Education & counselling of persons at risk on ways to adopt safer sexual behaviour.

11. State True/False with explanation.

(a) Abortions could happen spontaneously too. (True/False)

(b) Infertility is defined as the inability to produce a viable offspring and is always due to abnormalities/defects in the female partner. (True/False)

(c) Complete lactation could help as a natural method of contraception. (True/False)

(d) Creating awareness about sex related aspects is an effective method to improve reproductive health of the people. (True/False)

Sol. (a) *True*. Spontaneous abortion is non-induced embryonic or foetal death or passage of products (the foetus, foetal membranes, and placenta) from the uterus of conception before 20 wk gestation. Due to internal factors like incompatibility, abortion could happen spontaneously. Chromosomal abnormalities are a direct cause of spontaneous abortion.

Note

Autosomal trisomy was the most commonly identified anomaly (52 percent), followed by polyploidy (21 percent) and monosomy X (13 percent) in spontaneous abortion. Most chromosomal abnormalities that result in spontaneous abortion are random events, such as maternal and paternal gametogenesis errors, dispermy, and non-disjunction.

(b) *False*. Infertility is due to abnormalities/defects in either male or female or both the partners.

(c) *True*. Complete lactation could help as a natural method of contraception. Lactation limited to period up to six months after parturition. Lactation acts as a temporary contraceptive method which takes advantage of the way in which breastfeeding naturally makes a woman much less likely to conceive. Whilst breastfeeding, the amount of oestrogen produced by a woman's body is reduced thereby reduce the process of ovulation (release of egg from Graafian follicle into the fallopian tubes).

Note

- *Combined hormonal contraceptives are not recommended for use in breastfeeding women until at least six months after childbirth, as using these methods whilst breastfeeding may interfere with breast milk production and also reduce the quality of breast milk.*
- *Breast feeding doesn't completely avoid to getting pregnant but the chance of getting pregnant is lower.*

(d) True. Creating awareness about sex-related aspects removes the myths and misconceptions about these problems.

12. Correct the following statements :

(a) Surgical methods of contraception prevent gamete formation.

(b) All sexually transmitted diseases are completely curable.

(c) Oral pills are very popular contraceptives among the rural women.

(d) In E. T. techniques, embryos are always transferred into the uterus.

Sol. (a) Surgical methods of contraception *prevent gamete transport & thereby prevent conception.*

(b) All sexually transmitted diseases (STDs) *are not completely curable.* Except for hepatitis-B, genital herpes and HIV infections, other STD diseases are completely curable if detected early and treated properly.

(c) Oral pill are very popular contraceptives among the *educated urban women.*

(d) In E.T. (embryo transfer) techniques, *embryos are not always transferred into the uterus.* Because, embryos with 8 blastomeres are transferred into fallopian tube and more than 8 blastomeres are transferred into the uterus.

5 Chapter PRINCIPLES OF INHERITANCE AND VARIATION

CHAPTER AT A GLANCE

- **Heredity** is a process of transmission of traits from parents to their offspring's either *via* asexual reproduction or sexual reproduction. These characteristics or traits are located on the chromosomes in the form of genes.
- Term genetics was first used by **W. Bateson** (1905).
- The two Mendelian factors which occur on the same locus in the two homologous chromosomes of an individual and control the expression of a character are called **alleles** or **allelomorphs.**
- The heterozygous organism produced after crossing to genetically different individuals is called **hybrid**.
- **Back cross** is a cross which is performed between hybrid and one of its parents. Back cross are used by animal and plant breeders to rapidly improve a breed/variety by making a useful gene (trait) homozygous.
- **Test cross** is a cross to know whether an individual is homozygous or heterozygous for dominant character. Test cross is crossing of offspring with unknown dominant phenotype with the individual homozygous recessive for the trait.
  - If unknown offspring is homozygous (TT), then crossing with dwarf recessive (tt) gives all Tall offspring *i.e.*, Tt.
  - If unknown offspring is heterozygous tall (Tt), then crossing with dwarf recessive (tt) results in 50% tall (Tt) and 50% dwarf (tt) progeny.
- **True breeding line** is the one that has undergone continuous self pollination, shows stable trait inheritance and expression for several generations.
- **Gregor Johann Mendel** is called the **Father of genetics**. His genetic experiments were conducted on garden pea, *Pisum sativum* in 1856 in the garden at the monastery.
- Mendel used the pea plant for his experiments because of the following reasons:
  - Life span of pea plant is short.
  - Flowers are self-pollinated.
  - Flowers were hermaphrodite as well as bisexual.
- Mendel **selected 14 ture-breeding pea-plant varieties**, as pairs which were similar except for one character with contrasting traits. Some of the contrasting traits selected were smooth or wrinkled seeds, yellow or green seeds, smooth or inflated pods, green or yellow pods and tall or dwarf plants.

- A cross where transmission of one character is studied is called **monohybrid cross.**
- **Law of dominance** states that only one factor expresses itself in F_1 generation and expression of both factors expresses in F_2 generation in the proportion of 3 : 1 ratio.
- **Law of segregation** established the fact that alleles do not blend and both the traits are recovered as such in F_2 generation.
- **Law of independent assortment** states that genes of different characters located in different pairs of chromosomes are independent of one another in their segregation during gamete formation.
  This law was proposed by Mendel based on the results of dihybrid crosses, where inheritance of two traits were considered simultaneously.
- **Incomplete dominance** is a phenomenon where two contrasting alleles are present together but neither of the alleles is dominant over other and the phenotype formed is intermediate of the two alleles.
- Incomplete dominance was **discovered by Correns** in inheritance of flower colour in dog-flower (Snapdragon or *Antirrhinum majus*).
- In *Mirabili's jalapa* (four O' clock), there are two types of flower colour in pure state-red & white. When the two types of plants are crossed the hybrid or plants of F_1 generation have pink flowers. If the latter are selfed, the plants of F_2 generation are of three types-red, pink & white flowered in the ratio of 1 : 2 : 1.
- In **codominance**, both the alleles of a gene are equally dominant *i.e.* the dominant character is not able to suppress the recessive character & thus both the characters appear side by side in F_1 hybrids. F_1 generation resembles both the parents. E.g., ABO blood group, sickle cell anaemia.
- **Multiple alleles** can be defined as a set of three, four, or more allelomorphic genes or alleles, which have arisen as a result of mutation of the normal gene & which occupy the same locus in the homologous chromosomes.
- The well known example of multiple allele in human is blood group, which also shows codominance.
- **Chromosomal theory of inheritance theory states** that Mendelian genes (factors) are located on chromosome and it is the chromosome that segregate and independently assort.
- **Walter Sutton and Theodore Boveri** (1902) noted that the behaviour of chromosomes was parallel to the behaviour of genes and used chromosome movement to explain Mendel's Laws.
- **T. H. Morgan** is popularly called as **father of experimental genetics**.
- **Linkage** may be defined as the relationship between genes on the same chromosome that causes them to be inherited together, therefore it will not result in variations among siblings. In linkage there is a tendency to maintain the parental gene recombination except for occasional crossovers.

- The rearrangements of linked genes due to crossing over is known as **recombination.**
- **Polygenic inheritance** is the inheritance of a characteristic that is controlled by more than one gene. It can produce unexpected phenotypes.
- In **pleiotropy**, single gene controls multiple phenotypic expression whereas one gene controls or affects the phenotypic expression in case of Mendelism.
- **Grasshopper** has XO type of sex determination in which males have only one chromosome besides autosomes whereas female has a pair of X chromosomes.
- **XO type of sex determination** also occurs in honeybees, in which both ♂ and ♀ are isogametic/homogametic.
- **WZ type of sex determination in birds**
  ♀ = WZ configuration, ♂ = WW
- In humans, females have two X chromosomes (symbolised as XX) & males have two different sex chromosomes (symbolised as X & Y).
- Genetic makeup of sperm determines sex of child in human.

MUTATION AND GENETIC DISORDERS

- Phenomenon that results in alteration of DNA sequence and consequently results in change in genotype and phenotype of an organism is called **mutation**.
- **Pedigree analysis** is the study of an inherited trait in a group of related individuals. It helps to determine the pattern and characteristics of the trait which includes its mode of inheritance, age of onset, and phenotypic variability.
- A **genetic disorder** is a disease that is caused by an abnormality in an individual's DNA.
- Genetic disorder may be grouped into two categories – **Mendelian disorders** & **chromosomal disorders**.
- **Examples of Mendelian disorders** are :
  - **Haemophilia :** It is an X linked recessive disease. It occurs due to deficiency of plasma thromboplastin or antihaemophilia globulin during which the exposed blood does not clot.
  - **Sickle cell anaemia :** It is an autosomal recessive trait. It is a blood disease where the RBCs becomes sickle shaped as compared to normal one. It is due to inheritance of defective allele coding for β-globin. It results in the transformation of Hb^A into Hb^{-S} in which glutamic acid is replaced by valine at 6th position in each of two β-chains of haemoglobin.
- **Chromosomal disorders** are of two types – **autosomal chromosomal changes** & **sex chromosomal changes.**
- Autosomal disorders are of two types – euploidy and aneuploidy.
- **Euploidy** is the numerical increase of chromosome from normal 2n to multiples of complete haploid set. It is more common in plants, rare in animals & absent in humans.

- **Aneuploidy** relates to variation in chromosomes number with respect to one or only a few chromosomes.
- Examples of autosomal disorders are – Down's syndrome, Klinefelter's syndrome, Turner's syndrome, Edward syndrome, Patau's syndrome.
  - **Down syndrome (trisomy of 21)** syndrom is characterised by rounded face, low IQ, mongloid features, folded eyelids, short & broad neck, etc.
  - **Klinefelter's Syndrome (trisomy of 'X' chromosome)** is caused due to the presence of an additional copy of X-chromosome resulting into a karyotype of 47, XXY. Such an individual has overall masculine development, however, the feminine development (development of breast, *i.e.,* Gynaecomastia) is also expressed. Such individuals are sterile.
  - **Turner's Syndrome (monosomy of 'X' chromosome)** is caused due to the absence of one of the X chromosomes, *i.e.,* 45 with XO, such females are sterile as ovaries are rudimentary besides other features including lack of other secondary sexual characters.
  - **Edwards's syndrome** is caused by having an extra chromosome 18 in some or all of the body's cells. It is characterised by a low birth weight and certain abnormal features. These include a small, abnormally shaped head; a small jaw and mouth; clenched fists with overlapping fingers; and heart, lung, kidney, intestine, and stomach defects.
  - **Patau's syndrome** is a congenital disorder in which there are three copies of chromosome 13, 14, or 15 instead of the usual two. This results in brain, heart, and kidney defects which are usually fatal soon after birth.

EXERCISE

1. Mention the advantages of selecting pea plant for experiment by Mendel.

Sol. Mendel conducted hybridisation experiments on garden pea (*Pisum sativum*) to explain the inheritance of characters from parents to offspring.

The *advantages of selected garden pea* for experiment by Mendel are:

(i) It is an annual plant with short life span and produces large number of seeds in one generation. It is therefore, possible to study several generations within short period.

(ii) The plant is grown easily and does not require after care except at the time of pollination.

(iii) There are many garden pea varieties with visible characters with contrasting traits such as tall or dwarf plants, round or wrinkled seeds, green or yellow pod, purple or white flowers, etc.

(iv) It produces many seeds in one generation.

(v) It produces bisexual flowers and reproduces sexually through self pollination. Thus, it is easier to get pure lines.

(vi) Pea plants can be easily cross pollinated artificially by preventing self pollination by emasculation, *i.e.*, removal of the stamens of the flowers before anther dehiscence.

2. Differentiate between the following –
(a) Dominance and Recessive **(b) Homozygous and Heterozygous**
(c) Monohybrid and Dihybrid

Sol. (a) Difference between dominance and recessive

S. No.	Dominance	Recessive
1.	It is a factor or allele that expresses itself even in the presence of its alternate allele, *i.e.*, heterozygous condition.	It is a factor or allele that expresses itself only in the absence of its alternate allele, *i.e.*, only in the presence of the same allele or homozygous condition.
2.	It is expressed both in homozygous and heterozygous conditions.	It remains masked by dominant allele in heterozygous condition.
3.	It is denoted by capital letter, e.g., T for tall height.	It is denoted by small letter, e.g., t for dwarf height.

(b) Difference between homozygous and heterozygous

S. No.	Homozygous	Heterozygous
1.	It is the condition or individual with same alleles (either dominant or recessive) of a gene, e.g., homozygous tall pea plant with TT and homozygous dwarf pea plant with tt.	It is the condition or individual with different alleles (both dominant and recessive) of a gene, e.g., heterozygous tall pea plant with Tt.
2.	Such individuals produce one type of gametes, e.g., individual with TT will produce all the gametes with T allele and individual with tt will produce all gametes with t allele.	Such individuals produce two or more types of gametes, e.g., heterozygous tall plant will produce two types of gametes, allele T containing gametes and allele t containing gametes.
3.	Homozygous individuals are true breeding for a particular trait, *i.e.*, they produce offspring with same phenotype and genotypes of selfing. E.g., TT will produce progeny with TT.	Heterozygous individuals are not true breeding, *i.e.*, they produce offspring with different genotypes and phenotypes on selfing. E.g., Tt will produce plants with three genotypes and phenotypes, TT (homozygous tall plants), Tt (heterozygous tall plants) and tt (homozygous dwarf plants).

(c) Difference between monohybrid and dihybrid

S. No.	Monohybrid	Dihybrid
1.	It is a cross involving two individuals differing in one pair of contrasting traits e.g., cross between tall pea plants and dwarf pea plants.	It is a cross involving two individuals differing in two pairs of contrasting traits e.g., cross between pea plants having round and yellow seeds and pea plants having wrinkled and green seeds.
2.	The phenotypic ratio in F_2 generation of a monohybrid cross is 3:1.	The phenotypic ratio in F_2 generation of a dihybrid cross is 9:3:3:1.
3.	The genotypic ratio in F_2 generation of a monohybrid cross is 1:2:1.	The genotypic ratio in F_2 generation of a dihybrid cross is 1:2:1:2:4:2:1:2:1.

3. **A diploid organism is heterozygous for 4 loci, how many types of gametes can be produced?**

Sol. The formula to calculate the number of gametes produced will be 2^n where n is the number of heterozygous pair of genes.

So, in a diploid organism heterozygous for 4 loci, $2^4 = 16$ gametes will be produced.

4. **Explain the Law of Dominance using a monohybrid cross.**

Sol. According to law of dominance, when a pair of factors or alleles controlling alternative traits is brought together in F_1 hybrid, only one expresses itself while the other remains unexpressed. The factor or allele which expresses itself is called dominant factor or allele and the factor which remains masked is called recessive factor or allele.

Mendel postulated this law based on his observation on monohybrid cross. In a monohybrid cross, a cross is made between individuals differing in one pair of contrasting traits for example, tall and dwarf height of a plant. Thc allele T controls the tall height and the allele t controls the dwarf height. On crossing a true breeding tall pea plant (TT) with a true breeding dwarf pea plant (tt), F_1 hybrids with Tt genotype are obtained. Such hybrids are tall; this shows allele T is dominant over allele t and the trait tall is dominant and dwarf trait is recessive.

This cross can be represented as follows:

Parents	Tall	×	Dwarf
Genotype	TT		tt
Gametes	T		t
F_1 generation		Tt (Tall)	

5. Define and design a test cross.

Sol. When an F_1 individual with dominant phenotype is crossed with the homozygous recessive parent, it is called test cross. Test cross helps in establishing hetero- or homo-zygosity of dominant trait.

Example of a test cross :

On crossing a F_1 individual with tall height with dwarf plant, if all tall plants are produced then F_1 plant is homozygous (TT). This can be represented as follows:

F_1 Generation	TT	×	tt
Gametes	T		t
Offspring		Tt All tall	

On crossing a F_1 individual with tall height with dwarf plant, if tall and dwarf plants are produced in 1:1 ratio then F_1 plant is heterozygous (Tt). This can be represented as follows:

F_1 × recessive parent

F_1 generation	Tt Tall	×	tt Dwarf
Gametes	T t		t t
Offspring	Tt Tt 2 tall		tt tt 2 dwarf

Ratio – 1 : 1

> ***Note***
>
> *In case hybrid is heterozygous for dominant trait, test cross ratio of monohybrid cross is 1:1 whereas test cross ratio of dihybrid cross is 1:1:1:1.*

6. Using a Punnett Square, workout the distribution of phenotypic features in the first filial generation after a cross between a homozygous female and a heterozygous male for a single locus.

Sol. Let's consider two alternate traits-tall and dwarf controlled by alleles, T and t, respectively to find the distribution of phenotypic features in first filial generation of a cross between a homozygous female and a heterozygous male. The female could be homozygous dominant or homozygous recessive. So, this cross follows two conditions:

Condition 1:

Parents TT (♀) × Tt (♂)

Gametes (T) (T) (T) (t)

F_1 generation

♂ \ ♀	T	T
T	TT (Tall)	TT (Tall)
t	Tt (Tall)	Tt (Tall)

From the punnett square, it is observed that

Phenotype = All tall

Genotype ratio = TT : Tt

2 : 2

or 1 : 1

Condition 2:

Parents tt (♀) (Dwarf) × Tt (♂) (Tall)

Gametes (t) (t) (T) (t)

F_1 generation

♂ \ ♀	**t**	**t**
T	Tt (Tall)	Tt (Tall)
t	Tt (Dwarf)	Tt (Dwarf)

From the punnett square, it is observed that
Phenotypic ratio = Tall : Dwarf = 1:1
Genotypic ratio = Tt : tt = 1:1

7. **When a cross is made between tall plant with yellow seeds (TtYy) and tall plant with green seed (Ttyy), what proportions of phenotype in the offspring could be expected to be**
   (a) tall and green.
   (b) dwarf and green.

Sol. A cross between tall plant with yellow seeds (TtYy) and tall plant with green seeds (Ttyy) is given below.

Parents → Tall Yellow × Tall Green
Genotype Tt Yy × Tt yy

♂ \ ♀	Ty	ty
TY	TTYy (Tall, yellow)	TtYy (Tall, yellow)
Ty	Ttyy (Tall, green)	Ttyy (Tall, green)
tY	TtYy (Tall, yellow)	ttYy (Dwarf, yellow)
ty	Ttyy (Tall, green)	ttyy (Dwarf, green)

From this cross, the proportion of phenotypes:
(a) Tall and green = 3/8
(b) Dwarf and green = 1/8

8. **Two heterozygous parents are crossed. If the two loci are linked what would be the distribution of phenotypic features in F_1 generation for a dihybrid cross?**

Sol. Linkage is the phenomenon in which two or more genes present on the same chromosome are inherited together and do no assort independently. Such genes are called linked genes.
Let's consider two linked genes A and B controlling dominant traits. As per question, the genotype heterozygous parents will be AaBb.
The result of the cross between two heterozygous parents (AaBb) is shown below.

Parents AaBb × AaBb

Gametes (AB) (ab) (AB) (ab)

	AB	**ab**
AB	AaBb (Dominant characters)	AaBb (Dominant characters)
ab	AaBb (Dominant characters)	aabb (Recessive characters)

9. Briefly mention the contribution of T.H. Morgan in genetics.

Sol. Thomas Hunt Morgan (1866-1945), an American geneticist, who is famous for his work on *Drosophila melanogaster* as research material. He received Nobel Prize in Physiology or Medicine in 1933 and is considered as "Father of experimental genetics".

His *contributions in genetics are as follows*:

(i) He gave experimental verification of the chromosomal theory of inheritance by working with the tiny fruit flies, *Drosophila melanogaster* as research material.

(ii) He worked on sex linked inheritance and reported a white eyed male *Drosophila* in a population of red eyed and proved that gene of eye colour is located on X chromosome.

(iii) The male passed its genes on X chromosomes to the daughter while the son gets genes on X chromosome from the female (mother). It is called criss-cross inheritance.

(iv) In 1910, he discovered linkage and distinguished linked and unlinked genes. Morgan and Castle (1911) proposed "Chromosome Theory of Linkage" showing that genes are located in the chromosomes and arranged in linear order.

(v) Morgan and his student, Sturtevant (1911) found that frequency of crossing over (recombination) between two linked genes is directly proportional to the distance between the two. 1% recombination is considered to be equal to 1 centiMorgan (cM) or 1 map unit.

10. What is pedigree analysis? Suggest how such an analysis, can be useful.

Sol. Pedigree is a chart or table showing the presence or absence of a trait within a family across generations. A series of symbols are used to represent different aspects of a pedigree.

- The analysis of pedigree to study the inheritance of a particular trait in several generations of a family is called *pedigree analysis*.
- *Pedigree analysis can be useful* in the following ways:
  (i) When studying any population when progeny data from several generations is limited.
  (ii) When studying species with a long generation time.
  (iii) It helps to shows the relationship within an extended family. It also indicates the harm which arises in a marriage between close relatives.
  (iv) It determines the mode of inheritance (dominant, recessive, etc.) of genetic diseases.
  (v) It can also be used in the clinical setting, such as genetic counselling sessions or genetic evaluations, or in genetic research.
  (vi) It also indicates that Mendel's principles are also applicable to human genetics with some modifications found out later like quantitative inheritance, sex linked characters and other linkages.

11. How is sex determined in human beings?

Sol.
- Sex determining mechanism in humans is XX-XY type.
- Humans have 23 pairs of chromosomes out of which 22 pairs of autosomes which are exactly same in both males and females and one pair of sex chromosomes which are different in both males and females. The human females have a pair of X chromosomes as sex chromosomes whereas males have an X and Y chromosomes as sex chromosomes.
- Males produce two types of gametes, 50% sperms carrying 22 autosomes and one X chromosome and 50% sperms carrying 22 autosomes and one Y chromosome. Thus, males are heterogametic. Females, however, produce only one type of ovum *i.e.*, with 22 autosomes and an X chromosome. Therefore, females are homogametic.
- There is an equal probability of fertilisation of the ovum with the sperm carrying either X or Y chromosome. If an ovum fertilises with a sperm carrying X chromosome, the zygote possesses 44 autosomes and a pair of X chromosomes. Such a zygote develops into a female (XX). If fertilisation of ovum with Y-chromosome carrying sperm occurs, zygote possesses 44 autosomes and one X and Y chromosomes and results into a male offspring.

Thus, in humans, it is the *genetic makeup of the sperm that determines the sex of the child*. It is also evident that in each pregnancy there is always 50 per cent probability of either a male or a female child.

12. A child has blood group O. If the father has blood group A and mother of blood group B, work out the genotypes of the parents and the possible genotypes of the other offspring.

Sol. The inheritance of blood group in humans is an example of multiple alleles and is controlled by gene I with three alleles I^A, I^B and i. Alleles I^A and I^B are co-dominant to each other and completely dominant over allele i. The blood group O results when the individual is homozygous recessive (ii). The child in question will have both the recessive alleles, when the parents are heterozygous. Thus, genotype of father with blood group A will be I^Ai and that of mother with blood group B will be I^Bi.

The results of this cross are as follows:

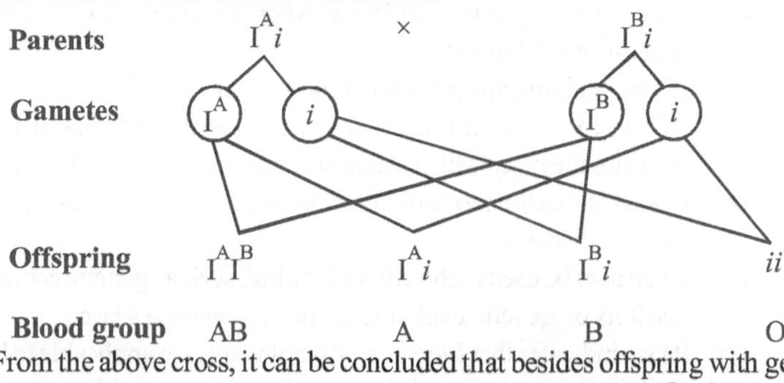

From the above cross, it can be concluded that besides offspring with genotype ii (blood group O), offspring with three other genotypes $I^A I^B$, $I^A i$ and $I^B i$ will also be produced.

13. Explain the following terms with example

(a) Co-dominance (b) Incomplete dominance

Sol. (a) Co-dominance

- It is the phenomenon in which a pair of alleles controlling two contrasting traits, when present together in an individual, lacks dominant-recessive relationship and both express themselves simultaneously. Thus, the individual resembles both the parents.
- ABO blood group is example co-dominance. ABO blood groups are controlled by the gene I which has three alleles I^A, I^B and *i*. The alleles I^A and I^B are completely dominant over *i*. But when I^A and I^B are present together, they both express and produce blood group AB; this is because of co-dominance.

(b) Incomplete dominance

- It is the phenomenon in which two alleles of a gene, when present together in F_1 hybrid, do not show dominace-recessiveness instead express them partially. As a result, F_1 hybrid does not resemble either of the parents and shows intermediate characteristic.
- The inheritance of flower colour in the dog flower (snapdragon or *Antirrhinum sp.*) is an example of incomplete dominance.
- When a true breeding red-flowered (RR) is crossed with a true breeding white-flowered plants (rr), the F_1 (Rr) was pink. On self pollination of F_1 plants, phenotypic ratio is 1 (RR) Red: 2 (Rr) Pink: 1 (rr) and white is obtained instead of 3:1 in F_2 generation.

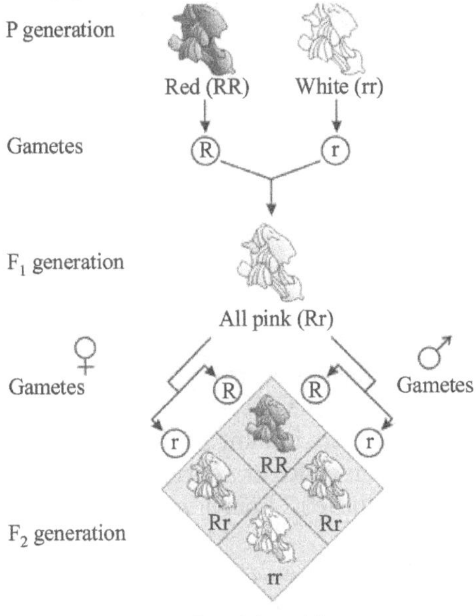

Phenotypic ratio : red : pink : white
1 : 2 : 1

Genotypic ratio : RR : Rr : rr
1 : 2 : 1

Fig.: Incomplete dominance in snapdragon

14. What is point mutation? Give one example.

Sol.
- Mutations arising due to change in single base pair of DNA is called *point mutation.*
- An *example of point mutation* is sickle cell anaemia. It results from single base substitution at the sixth codon of the beta globin gene from GAG to GUG. This base substitution results in substitution of Glutamic acid (Glu) by Valine (Val) at the sixth position of the beta globin chain of the haemoglobin molecule. The mutant haemoglobin molecule undergoes polymerisation under low oxygen tension causing the change in the shape of the RBC from biconcave disc to elongated sickle like structure.

15. Who had proposed the chromosomal theory of the inheritance?

Sol.
- *Sutton and Boveri* in 1902 *proposed the chromosomal theory of the inheritance.* They found parallelism in the behaviour of chromosomes and genes. They used chromosome movement to explain Mendel's laws.
- This theory believes that chromosomes are vehicles of Mendelian factors or genes. This is the chromosomes which segregate and assort independently during transmission from one generation to the next. It is the separation of a pair of chromosomes which leads to the segragation of a pair of factors present on them.
- Experimental verification of this theory was given by T.H. Morgan and his colleagues.

16. Mention any two autosomal genetic disorders with their symptoms.

Sol. Autosomal genetic disorders result from the mutation in genes present on autosomes. Males and females are equally affected with these disorders. *Two examples of autosomal genetic disorders* in humans are as follows:

(i) **Sickle cell anaemia**

- This is an autosome linked recessive trait that affects the red blood cell. It is controlled by a single pair of allele, Hb^A and Hb^S. Out of the three possible genotypes, only homozygous individuals for Hb^S (Hb^SHb^S) show the diseased phenotype whereas heterozygous (Hb^AHb^S) individuals appear apparently unaffected but they are carrier of the disease.
- It can be transmitted from parents carrier for the gene (or heterozygous) to the offspring.
- In this disorder, mutant haemoglobin molecule undergoes polymerisation under low oxygen tension causing the change in the shape of the RBC from biconcave disc to elongated sickle like structure.
- *Symptoms of this disorders* are anaemia due to early death of sickle-shaped cells, painful swelling of hands and feet, fatigue or or extreme tiredness; and jaundice. Over time, sickle cell disease can lead to complications such as infections, delayed growth, and episodes of pain, called pain crises.

(ii) **Phenylketonuria**

- This is inborn error of metabolism and also inherited as the autosomal recessive trait. This will result in decreased metabolism of amino acid phenylalanine. The affected individual lacks an enzyme (phenylalanine hydroxylase) that converts the amino acid phenylalanine into tyrosine. As a result, phenylalanine is accumulated and converted into phenylpyruvic acid and other derivatives. These are also excreted through urine because of its poor absorption by kidney.
- *Symptoms of this disorder* include seizures, skin rashes (eczema), abnormally small head (microcephaly), delayed development, behavioural, emotional and social problems, psychiatric disorders, etc.

Chapter 6

MOLECULAR BASIS OF INHERITANCE

CHAPTER AT A GLANCE

- **Genetic material** is that substance which not only controls the formation and expression of traits in an organism but can replicate & pass from a cell to its daughter cell or from one generation to another.
- **DNA** (deoxyribonucleic acid) and **RNA** (ribonucleic acid) are two types of nucleic acids, found in living systems.

DEOXYRIBONUCLEIC ACID (DNA)

- DNA is the hereditary material in humans and almost all other organisms.
- Most DNA is located in the cell nucleus (where it is called nuclear DNA), but a small amount of DNA can also be found in the mitochondria (where it is called mitochondrial DNA or mtDNA).
- DNA consists of a nitrogenous base, pentose sugar and a phosphate group.
- A nucleotide is a basic building block of DNA.
- A nitrogenous base is attached to the pentose sugar by an N-glycosidic linkage to form a nucleoside, *i.e.*, Nucleoside =Nitrogen base + Pentose sugar.
- In 1953, **James Watson and Francis** revealed the **'double helix' model of the structure of DNA**, based on X-ray diffraction data from Maurice Wilkins and Rosalind Franklin.
- It consists of two polynucleotide chains where the sugar and phosphate group form the backbone and the nitrogenous bases project inside the helix.
- The two polynucleotide chains have anti-parallel polarity i.e. if one strand has $5' \rightarrow 3'$ polarity, the other strand has $3' \rightarrow 5'$ polarity.
- Nitrogenous base are of two types – **purines** (9 membered double rings with nitrogen at 1, 3, 7 & 9th positions) and **pyrimidines** (6 membered rings with nitrogen at 1 and 3rd position).
- Purines are of **two types** – adenine (A) and guanine (G) and pyrimidines are of **three types** – thymine (T), cytosine (C) and uracil (U).
- A characteristics that differentiate DNA from RNA is that DNA contains all of the nitrogen bases except uracil and RNA contains all of the nitrogen bases except thymine.
- Pentose sugar is **deoxyribose** in DNA and **ribose in RNA**.
- DNA is composed of 2 strands wound around each other to form a double helix, with base inside and sugar phosphate backbone on outside.

- 2 DNA strands are organised in antiparallel and complementary arrangement [*i.e.,* 2 strands run in opposite orientation (one in 5' – 3' and allies in 3' – 5')].
- A = T, G ≡ C is called **complementary base pairing** that makes sequencing possible if template strand sequence is known.
- **Erwin Chargaff** (1950) found that purine and pyrimidine contents of DNA are equal.
- DNA of bacteria such as *E.coli* is a circular double stranded molecule which contain 4.6 million base pairs.
- **Eukaryotic DNA** is organised into bead structure called **nucleosome**.
- Negatively charged DNA is wrapped around this positively charged histone octamer to form nucleosome.
- On the basis of packaging, chromatin is classified into 2 types – euchromatin and heterochromatin.
  - **Euchromatin** is transcriptionally active, loosely packed, rich in gene concentration, lightly stained.
  - **Heterochromatin** is transcriptionally inactive, densely packed, darkly stained.
- Establishment of DNA as genetic material by Griffith who carried out experiment with *Streptococcus pneumoniae* (bacterium causing pneumonia) which is used to infect mice.
- **Hershey & Chase** (1962) discovered that DNA is the genetic material of bacteriophage.
- **DNA replication or DNA synthesis** is the process of copying a double stranded DNA prior to cell division.
- Replication of DNA is found to be semiconservative and its experimental proof has been provided by **Meselson** and **Stahl in 1958.**
- DNA replication **occurs during S phase of cell cycle** and require template and DNA polymerase along with primer.
- DNA replication begins at a specific site called **ori (origin)** which has recognition site for DNA polymerase, which also provides site for attachment of RNA primer.
- The enzyme which form RNA from DNA are called RNA polymerase. The synthesis of RNA primer is brought about by enzyme primase.
- In bacterial chromosome, replication starts at a single origin and both strands of a double helix serve as template for DNA synthesis which proceeds outwards in both directions from single origin (*i.e.,* it is bidirectional).
- dsDNA is antiparallel, one strand runs in 5'-3' direction and its complementary runs in 3'-5'. New DNA strand is made against each template strand. DNA polymerase makes DNA only in 5'-3' direction. So are template strand with 3'-5' orientation, new DNA strand is made in continuous piece in correct 5'-3' direction. This DNA is called **leading strand**.

- On template strand which has 5' → 3' orientation, DNA polymerase synthesizes short pairs of new DNA (about 1000 nucleotides long) in 5' → 3' direction and then joins these piece together. These small fragments are called **okazaki fragments** and new DNA strand made in this **discontinuous manner** is called **lagging strand**. Okazaki fragments are joined by means of DNA ligase.

RIBONUCLEI ACID (RNA)

- RNA is a vital molecule with a long chain of nucleotides. It is a first genetic material. A nucleotide chain comprises a phosphate, a ribose sugar, and nitrogenous base.
- RNA acts as a catalyst and as a genetic material.
- RNA is a non hereditary nucleic acid except in some viruses (retro viruses).
- On the basis of molecular size & function, three forms of non genetic RNA are–
  - **mRNA (messenger RNA)** – provides template for translation.
  - **tRNA (transfer RNA)** – brings aminoacids and reads genetic code.
  - **rRNA (ribosomal RNA)** – structural and catalytic role during translation.
- **RNA processing : In prokaryotes**, mRNA transcribed from protein coding genes requires no modification prior to translation. In fact, many mRNA molecules begin to translate even before RNA synthesis has finished. **Ribosomal RNA** (rRNA) and **transfer RNA** (tRNA) are synthesised as precursor molecule that do not require **post-transcriptional processing**.
- RNA transcription requires enzyme RNA polymerase, DNA template, all four types of ribonucleoside triphosphates (ATP, GTP, CTP & UTP), divalent metal ions Mg^{2+} or Mn^{2+} as cofactor, rho (ρ) factor etc.
- RNA polymerase can initiate transcription at specific DNA sequences known as promoters. It then produces an RNA chain which is complementary to the DNA strand used as template.

GENETIC CODE AND PROTEIN SYNTHESIS

- **Genetic code** is defined as a relationship between the sequence of amino acids in a nucleotide chain of mRNA or DNA and amino acid in a polypeptide chain.
- Triplet nature of genetic code was proposed by **F.H.C.Crick**.
- **Nirenberg** gave the first experimental proof for triplet code.
- **UGA, UAG and UAA** are **nonsense codon** which do not code for any amino acid.
- **Wobble hypothesis** explains why multiple codons can code for a single amino acid. This hypothesis states that the third position (3') of the codon on mRNA and the first position (5') of the anticodon on tRNA are bound less tightly than the other pair and therefore unusual base combination
- The characteristics of the genetic code are degeneracy of genetic code, non-overlapping, universality, triplet in nature, comma-less, non-ambiguous.
- **Protein synthesis** is a process of creating protein molecules. It involves amino acid synthesis, transcription, and translation.

- Process of copying genetic information from one strand of DNA to RNA is called **transcription.**
- The strand of DNA with polarity 3' → 5' act as **template** strand and the DNA strand with polarity 5' → 3' act as **coding strand.**
- Transcription is carried out by DNA dependent RNA polymerase.
- **Transcription** unit is the segment of deoxyribonucleic acid between the sites of initiation & termination of transcription.
- **Transcription and translation** takes place in same compartment (there is no separate cytosol and nucleus in bacteria). So transcription and translation are coupled in bacteria where as in **eukaryotes** transcription and translation occur in nucleus and cytosol respectively and thus compartmentalised.
- Transfer of genetic information from a polymer of nucleotides to a polymer of amino acids is called **translation**.. This is accomplished with the help of genetic code which is row of three consecutive nucleotides – coding for 20 amino acids.
- Codon exists on mRNA, corresponding anticodon on tRNA and protein synthesis and elongation occurs in rRNA.
- tRNA is intermediate between reading of codons on mRNA and formation of amino acid chain for protein.
- The **main step in protein synthesis** are activation, initiation, elongation & termination of polypeptide chain.

REGULATION OF GENE EXPRESSION

- **Gene expression** is the mechanism at the molecular level by which a gene is able to express itself in the phenotype of an organisms.
- In eukaryotes, the regulation could be exerted at–
  (i) Transcriptional level (formation of primary transcript).
  (ii) Processing level (RNA splicing) level.
  (iii) Transport of mRNA from nucleus to cytoplasm.
  (iv) Translational level.
- One of the best studied example of gene expression is **lac operon.**
- Model of lac operon was suggested by **Jacob** and **Monod** in 1961.
- In lac operon, a polycistronic structural gene is regulated by a common **promoter & regulatory genes.**
- Structural genes produces 3 enzymes for the degradation of lactose to glucose & galactose.
- **Operator gene :** DNA sequence that regulates transcription of the structural genes.
- **Regulator gene :** Encodes a protein that recognizes operon sequence.
- Regulation of the operon by repressor is called as **negative regulation** as it decreases expression of structural gene.
- **Positive control** of gene expression is when the regulatory protein binds to DNA and increases rate of transcription. In this case the regulating protein is called an activator.

HUMAN GENOME PROJECT AND DNA FINGERPRINTING

- **Human Genome Project** established whole genome of human with the help of genetic engineering techniques, cloning techniques and bioinformatics.
- **DNA fingerprinting** is a technique for identifying individuals, generally using repeated sequences (repetitive DNA) in the human genome that produces a pattern of band that is unique for every individual.
- DNA technique has following steps:
  - Isolation of DNA and digestion of DNA by restriction endonucleases.
  - Separation of DNA fragments by (gel) electrophoresis and transferring (blotting) of separated DNA fragments to synthetic membrane or nitrocellulose or nylon.
  - Hybridisation using VNTR probe and detection of hybridised DNA fragments by autoradiography.
  - Matching the banding pattern so obtained with that of relative.

EXERCISE

1. Group the following as nitrogenous bases and nucleosides: Adenine, Cytidine, Thymine, Guanosine, Uracil and Cytosine.

Sol. Nitrogenous bases are Adenine, Uracil, Cytosine, Thymine. Nucleosides (Nitrogenous base + sugar) are Cytidine and Guanosine.

2. If a double stranded DNA has 20 per cent of cytosine, calculate the per cent of adenine in the DNA.

> ***Hints***
>
> *Apply Chargaff's rule.*

Sol. According to Chargaff's rule, in a double-stranded DNA, the ratios between cytosine and guanine & adenine and thymine are constant and equals one, *i.e.*, number of cytosine is equal to the number of guanine and the number of adenine is equal to number of thymine.

So, % C = % G

% T = % A

As per question, double-stranded DNA has 20% cytosine then according to Chargaff's rule, it will have 20% guanine.

Total percentage of G + C content = 20% + 20% = 40%

Total percentage of A + T content = 100% – 40% = 60%

Since adenine and thymine are present in equal number, content of adenine will be 30%.

3. **If the sequence of one strand of DNA is written as follows:**
5′-ATGCATGCATGCATGCATGCATGCATGC-3′
Write down the sequence of complementary strand in 5′→3′ direction.

Sol. According to complementary base pairing property of DNA, adenine present in one DNA strand always base pairs with thymine of the complementary strand and guanine in a DNA strand always base pairs with cytosine of the complementary strand and *vice versa*.
If the sequence of one DNA strand is:
5'-ATGCATGCATGCATGCATGCATGCATGC-3'
Since two strands in a double-stranded DNA are antiparallel, the sequence of complementary strand in 3' to 5' direction will be:
3'-TACGTACGTACGTACGTACGTACGTACG-5'
The sequence of complementary strand in 5' to 3' direction will be:
5'-GCATGCATGCATGCATGCATGCATGCAT-3'

4. **If the sequence of the coding strand in a transcription unit is written as follows:**
5′-ATGCATGCATGCATGCATGCATGCATGC-3′
Write down the sequence of mRNA.

Sol. Coding strand in a transcription unit is the DNA strand with polarity 5' → 3' and does not code for any protein. It has the base sequence same as RNA except thymine at the place of uracil.
If the sequence of coding strand is:
5'-ATGCATGCATGCATGCATGCATGCATGC-3'
The *sequence of mRNA will be*:
5'-AUGCAUGCAUGCAUGCAUGCAUGCAUGC-3'

5. **Which property of DNA double helix led Watson and Crick to hypothesise semi-conservative mode of DNA replication? Explain.**

Sol. Watson and Crick observed that *the nitrogenous bases are in complementary pairing in two strands of double helix of DNA molecule*. Such an arrangement of DNA molecule led them to *hypothesise the semiconservative mode of replication of DNA*.
During DNA replication, the two DNA strands separate and act as a template for the synthesis of new complementary strands. The sequence of newly synthesised DNA is determined by the sequence of bases on the template strand based on complementary base pairing rule. After the completion of replication, each daughter DNA molecule has one parental and one newly synthesised strand. Since only one parental strand is present from one generation to the next, this mode of replication is called semiconservative.

6. Depending upon the chemical nature of the template (DNA or RNA) and the nature of nucleic acids synthesised from it (DNA or RNA), list the types of nucleic acid polymerases.

Sol. Different types of nucleic acid polymerases are as follows:

Nucleic acid polymerase	Template	Nucleic acid synthesised
DNA-dependent DNA polymerase	DNA	DNA
DNA-dependent RNA polymerase	DNA	RNA
RNA-dependent DNA polymerase (Reverse transcriptase)	RNA	cDNA

7. How did Hershey and Chase differentiate between DNA and protein in their experiment while proving that DNA is the genetic material?

Sol. Alfred Hershey and Martha Chase (1952) worked with viruses that infect bacteria called bacteriophages. In 1952, they chose a bacteriophage known as T_2 as their experimental material to prove that DNA is the genetic material. To differentiation between DNA and protein they grew some viruses on a medium that contained radioactive phosphorus (^{32}p) and some others on medium that contained radioactive sulphur (^{35}s). Viruses grown in the presence of radioactive phosphorus contained radioactive DNA but not radioactive protein because DNA contains phosphorus containing nucleotides but protein does not. Similarly, viruses grown on radioactive sulphur contained radioactive protein but not radioactive DNA because DNA does not contain sulphur and proteins contain sulphur containing amino acids.

Radioactive phages were allowed to attach to *E. coli* bacteria. Then, as the infection proceeded, the viral coats were removed from the bacteria by agitating them in a blender. The virus particles were separated from the bacteria by spinning them in a centrifuge.

Bacteria which was infected with viruses that had radioactive DNA were radioactive, indicating that DNA was the material that passed from the virus to the bacteria. Bacteria that were infected with viruses that had radioactive proteins were not radioactive. This indicates that proteins did not enter the bacteria from the viruses. DNA is therefore the genetic material that is passed from virus to bacteria.

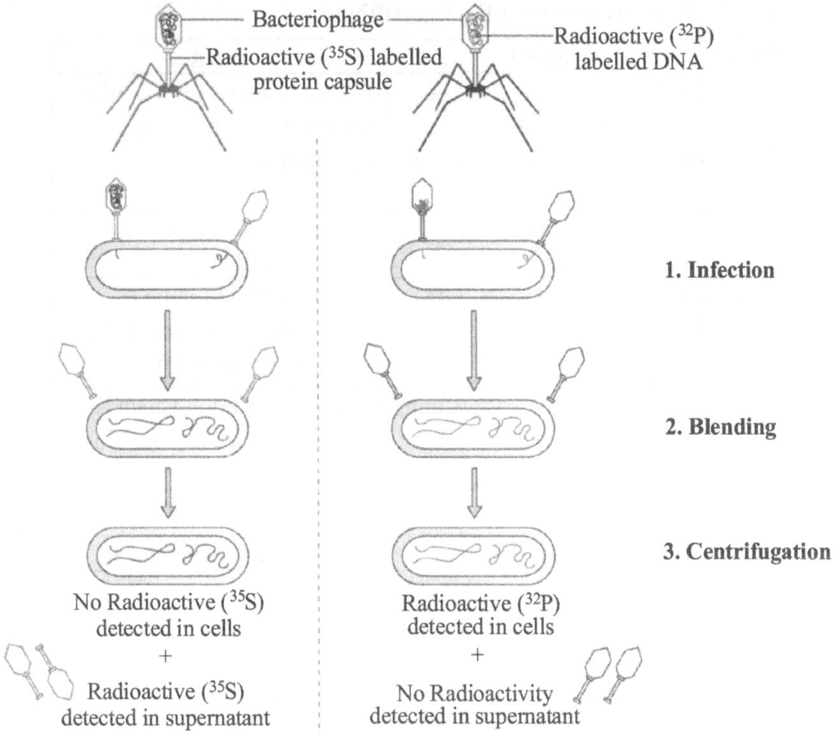

Fig.: The Harshey and Chase experiment

8. **Differentiate between the followings:**
   (a) **Repetitive DNA and Satellite DNA**
   (b) **mRNA and tRNA**
   (c) **Template strand and Coding strand**

Sol. (a) Differences between repetitive DNA and satellite DNA

S.No.	Repetitive DNA	Satellite DNA
1.	Repetitive DNA is the non-coding DNA with multiple copies of identical sequences, which may be interspersed or arranged in tandem.	Satellite DNA is a type of repetitive DNA that comprises of short sequences present as head-to-tail tandem repeats.
2.	It is of two types - tandem repetitive sequences (known as satellite DNA) and the interspersed repeats.	It is classified into the macrosatellites, minisatellites and microsatellites.

(b) Differences between mRNA and tRNA

S.No.	mRNA	tRNA
1.	mRNA or messenger RNA carries the genetic information to ribosomes for the synthesis of protein.	tRNA or transfer RNA carries amino acids to the site of protein synthesis, *i.e.*, ribosomes.
2.	It is synthesised by RNA polymerase II.	It is synthesised by RNA polymerase III.
3.	It is a linear molecule.	Its secondary structure is clover leaf like and inverted L-shaped in compact form.
4.	It carries genetic information in the form of codons.	It carries anticodon which is complementary to a codon on mRNA.

(c) Differences between template strand and coding strand

S.No.	Template strand	Coding strand
1.	Template strand is a DNA strand with polarity 3'→5'.	Coding strand is a DNA strand with polarity 5'→3'.
2.	It is also called antisense strand.	It is also called sense strand.
3.	It serves as a template for the synthesis of mRNA during transcription.	It does not code for mRNA.
4.	This strand is complementary to mRNA synthesised from it.	This strand has the same sequence as mRNA except for uracil in place of thymine.

9. List two essential roles of ribosome during translation.

Sol. A ribosome is a compact ribonucleoprotein particle which has two subunits, one large subunit and one small subunit. They associate with different mRNAs for the synthesis of different polypeptides.

Ribosome perform the following *essential roles during protein synthesis or translation*:

(i) The ribosome provides the binding site for mRNA in small subunit and two binding sites for subsequent amino acids in the large subunit and thus, be close enough to each other for the formation of a peptide bond. It also moves along mRNA by three nucleotides each time to add amino acids sequentially to the growing polypeptide. In this way, it provides an environment in which recognition between a codon of mRNA and anticodon of tRNA occurs and aminoacyl-tRNAs add amino acids to the growing chain in response to the corresponding triplet codons.

(ii) The ribosome also acts as a catalyst. The large subunit of ribosome has peptidyl transferase activity for the formation of peptide bond between two amino acids. This activity is associated with 23S rRNA in large subunit of ribosome of bacteria so this enzyme is a ribozyme.

10. In the medium where *E. coli* was growing, lactose was added, which induced the *lac* operon. Then, why does *lac* operon shut down some time after addition of lactose in the medium?

Sol. *Lac* operon is an operon in bacteria which contains structural genes responsible for metabolism of lactose. It consists of one regulatory gene, gene *lac i* and three structural genes, *lac z*, *lac y* and *lac a* (which codes for three enzymes β-galactosidase, permease and transacetylase respectively). Lactose is the substrate for the enzyme β-galactosidase and it regulates switching on and off of the operon. Hence, it is called inducer. In the absence of a preferred carbon source such as glucose, if lactose is provided in the growth medium of the bacteria, the lactose is transported into the cells through the action of permease. Lactose binds to the repressor and prevents its binding to operator. This allows RNA polymerase access to the promoter and transcription of structural genes proceeds leading to the formation of β-galactosidase. This enzyme breaks down the lactose into glucose and galactose.

After sometime, *lac operon shuts down due to the following reasons*:

(i) As inducer is completely metabolised, lactose is not available to inactivate repressor. This results in binding of repressor to the operator gene and in turn, preventing RNA polymerase from transcribing the operon. Hence, the transcription is stopped and operon is switched off.

(ii) *Lac* operon cannot be switched on by lactose due to accumulation of glucose which is preferred energy source than lactose.

11. Explain (in one or two lines) the function of the followings:

(a) Promoter (b) tRNA (c) Exons

Sol. (a) Promoter: Promoter is one of the three regions of transcription unit located towards 5' end of the structural gene. It is a DNA sequence that provides binding site for RNA polymerase to initiate transcription. Also, the position of a promoter in a transcription unit defines the template and coding strands.

(b) tRNA: tRNA or transfer RNA is a 75 to 85 long ribonucleic acid folded to form a secondary structure shaped like a cloverleaf. Each tRNA molecule has an anticodon loop that has bases complementary to the code, and an amino acid acceptor end to which it binds to amino acids. Each tRNA has only one type of anticodon and attaches to a specific amino acid. Its function is to bind to an activated amino acid, transfer it from cellular pool to ribosomes where tRNA binds to correct codon in mRNA and helps assemble amino acids into polypeptides.

(c) Exons: Exons are coding sequences interrupted by non-coding sequences (called introns) in the split genes of eukaryotes. Introns are removed and exons are joined to produce functional RNA by splicing. The exons in functional mRNA are transcribed into functional polypeptide.

12. Why is the Human genome project called a mega project?

Sol. Human genome project aimed to sequence every base in human genome. It was a 13-year project coordinated by the U.S. Department of Energy and the National Institute of Health. The project was completed in 2003.

It was a *mega project due to the following reasons*:

(i) *Large size of human genome and high invested cost of sequencing*: Human genome is said to have approximately 3×10^9 bp and the total estimated cost of the project would be approximately 9 billion US dollars, and if the cost of sequencing required is US $ 3 per bp (the estimated cost in the beginning).

(ii) *Requirement of high speed computational devices for data storage*: The enormous amount of data would be expected to generate from DNA sequencing from a single human cell. This necessitated the use of high speed computational devices for data storage and retrieval, and analysis. HGP was closely associated with the rapid development of a new area in biology called bioinformatics.

13. What is DNA fingerprinting? Mention its application.

Sol.
- *DNA fingerprinting* is a technique used to identify individuals based on the differences in some specific regions in DNA sequence called as repetitive DNA. It works on the principle of polymorphism in DNA sequences. This technique was initially developed by Sir Alec Jeffreys who discovered that certain regions of DNA showed variations in the number of tandem repeats known as variable number of tandem repeats (VNTRs). He used a satellite DNA as probe that shows very high degree of polymorphism.
- *Application of DNA fingerprinting:*

  (i) It can be applied in forensic science to identify an individual in criminal and civil cases.

  (ii) DNA fingerprinting is the basis of paternity testing, in case of disputes.

  (iii) It is used to identify genes connected with hereditary diseases.

  (iv) It is used to identify and protect the commercial varieties of crops and livestock.

  (v) It finds its application in evolutionary biology where it is used to find out the evolutionary history of an organism and trace out the linkages between groups of various organisms.

14. Briefly describe the following:

(a) Transcription

(b) Polymorphism

(c) Translation

(d) Bioinformatics

Sol. (a) Transcription

- It is the process in which genetic information from DNA is copied into RNA.
- In transcription, only a segment of DNA is copied into RNA. The segment of DNA that codes for RNA is called transcription unit. A transcription unit in DNA has three regions namely promoter, structural gene and a terminator. The promoter and terminator flank the structural gene in a transcription unit. The promoter is a DNA sequence that provides binding site for RNA polymerase. The terminator defines the end of the process of transcription. Also during transcription, one of the strands of DNA acts a template to direct the synthesis of complementary RNA.
- RNA is transcribed from DNA strand with polarity $3' \rightarrow 5'$ by the enzyme DNA-dependent RNA polymerase in $5' \rightarrow 3'$ direction using ribonucleotides.
- The process of transcription completes in three steps: initiation, elongation and termination. During initiation, RNA polymerase binds to promoter and initiates transcription (initiation). It uses nucleoside triphosphates as substrate.

(b) Polymorphism

- Polymorphism refers to the variation at genetic level arising due to mutations.
- DNA polymorphism is an inheritable mutation observed in a population at high frequency. The probability of such variation is higher in non-coding DNA sequence as mutations in these sequences may not have any immediate effect or impact in an individual's reproductive ability.
- These mutations keep on accumulating generation after generation, and form one of the bases of variability or polymorphism. There is a variety of different types of polymorphisms ranging from single nucleotide change to very large scale changes. For evolution and speciation, such polymorphisms play very important role.
- Polymorphism in DNA sequence also forms the basis of genetic mapping of human genome as well as of DNA fingerprinting.

(c) Translation

- Translation is the process of protein synthesis from mRNA. The mRNA provides the template, tRNA brings amino acids and reads the genetic code, and rRNAs play structural and catalytic role during translation.
- During translation, amino acids are polymerised to form a polypeptide. The order and sequence of amino acids in a polypeptide are defined by the sequence of bases in the mRNA.
- The steps in translation are:
  (i) The ribosome binds to mRNA at a specific area.
  (ii) The ribosome starts matching tRNA anticodon sequences to the mRNA codon sequence.
  (iii) Each time a new tRNA comes into the ribosome, the amino acid that it was carrying gets added to the elongating polypeptide chain. The ribosome continues until it hits a stop sequence, then it releases the polypeptide and the mRNA.
  (iv) The polypeptide forms into its native shape and starts acting as a functional protein in the cell.

Note

In bacteria, transcription and translation take place in the same compartment and many times the translation can begin much before the mRNA is fully transcribed because there is no separation of cytosol from nucleus in bacteria. In contrast, in eukaryotes, transcription takes place in nucleus and translation occurs in cytoplasm.

(d) Bioinformatics

- Bioinformatics is an interdisciplinary field mainly involving molecular biology and genetics, computer science, mathematics, and statistics.
- This field develops methods and software tools for understanding biological data. It helps to analyse and compare protein sequences, search for genes, assemble genomes, compare species based on their genetic material, forecast protein structures and find active parts of proteins, analyse gene expression, and inverse engineer genetic networks.
- It also helps to relate the genome to its phenotype and can trace evolution back to its roots to find adaptations and changes in the organisms.

Chapter 7

EVOLUTION

CHAPTER AT A GLANCE

- **Evolution** is the formation of newer types of organisms from the pre-existing ones through modification.

ORIGIN OF LIFE

- **Origin of life** is the process by which living organisms developed from inanimate matter, which is generally thought to have occurred on Earth between 3500 to 4000 millions years ago.
- Earth originated **4600 million year ago**.
- Life appeared 3.7 billion years ago. This is indicated by the discovery of microfossils of cyanobacteria like organisms.
- There was **no atmosphere on early earth**.
- There are **various theories** which explain the phenomenon of origin of life. A few of them were only assumptions while others were based on scientific grounds. These theories are – Theory of special creation, Theory of spontaneous generation or Abiogenesis, Theory of biogenesis, and Oparin Haldane theory.
- **Oparin and Haldane** proposed that the first form of life could have come from pre-existing non-living organic molecules (**e.g.,** RNA, protein etc.) and that formation of life was preceeded by chemical evolution, *i.e.*, formation of diverse organic molecules from inorganic constituents.
- **Oparin – Haldane theory** was supported experimentally by **Miller-Urey** experiment in 1953 with the help of simulation experiments. Miller & Urey tried to create conditions existing in primitive atmosphere – in **spark discharge apparatus** – a large flask containing mixture of CH_4, NH_3, H_2 and H_2O with electric source and boiling of water for a week. They observed formation of amino acids.
- The Miller-Urey experiment provided the first evidence that organic molecules needed for life could be formed from inorganic components.
- **Haldane** coined the term **'prebiotic soup'**, and this became a powerful symbol of the Oparin-Haldane view of the origin of life.
- Prebiotic soup is also called **hot dilute soup**.
- Oparin postulated the spontaneous appearance of structures called **coacervates**.
- The first prokaryotes were **anaerobes and chemoheterotrophs**.
- Atmosphere becomes richer in oxygen **due to photoautotrophs**.

1. Free atoms – H, C, N, O, etc.
   ↓
2. Origin of simple inorganic compounds – H_2, H_2O, NH_3, etc.
   ↓
3. Origin of early organic compounds – CH_4, HCN, etc
   ↓
4. Origin of simple organic compounds – Simple sugars, fatty acids, glycerol, amino acids, nitrogenous bases (purines and pyrimidines)
   ↓
5. Origin of complex organic compounds – Polysaccharides, fat, proteins, nucleotides, nucleic acids
   ↓
6. Origin of coacervates – Aggregates of complex organic molecules capable of growth and division
   ↓
7. Eobiont (proto cells) – Clusters of nucleoproteins and other substances capable of synthesis, replication, mutation and adaptation
   ↓
8. Prokaryotes – Without organised nucleus, chemoheterotrophs and anaerobic.
   ↓
9. Eukaryotes – With well organised nucleus

Flow chart : Main steps in origin of life according to Modern theory of origin of life

THEORIES OF EVOLUTION

- Darwin published his observations and conclusions regarding evolution in the book "Origin of Species" in 1859.
- Darwin proposed the **theory of evolution by natural selection**. According to this theory, individuals that are better adapted to their environment survive and reproduce more successfully than less well adapted individuals.
- Darwin travelled round the world in ship H.M.S. Beagle for 5 years and during journey, he noted a huge variety and remarkable similarity between organisms and their wonderful adaptation to environment and proposed the following factors:
  - Rapid multiplication
  - Limited environmental resources
  - Struggle for existence
  - Variation
  - Natural selection
  - Survival of fittest
  - Inheritance of useful variation
  - Formation of new species

- Due to limited space and food, the following competition **occurs for struggle for existence.**
  - **Intraspecific :** Between individuals of same species.
  - **Interspecific :** Between individuals of different species.
  - **Environmental :** Natural calamites like flood, drought.
- The **mutation theory** was put forward by **Hugo de vries** to explain the mechanism of evolution.
- **Features of mutation theory** are–
  - Mutation (Sudden, discontinuous, inheritable, genetic variation) form raw material for evolution.
  - It appears suddenly and produces effect immediately.
  - Mutants are different from parents.
  - Mutations are recurring, random, inheritable.
  - Collection of mutated forms leads to evolution.
- The mutation observed by de Vries in *Oenothera Lamarckiana* was chromosomal number variant.
- **Genetic equilibrium (Hardy Weinberg law)** states that "both gene frequency and genotype frequency" will remain constant from generation to generation in an infinitely large interbreeding population in which mating is random and no selection, migration or mutation occurs.
- **Genetic drift** refers to chance elimination of gene(s) of certain traits when a section of population migrates or dies of natural calamity. It eliminates certain alleles and fixes other alleles.
- Members of a population might enter a new population and interbreed there. They will add new allels to the local gene pool of the host population. This is called **gene migration**. (It may be in case of inter-specific fertile cross).
- **Types of selection**
  - **Stabilising selection :** Intermediate characteristics are favoured.

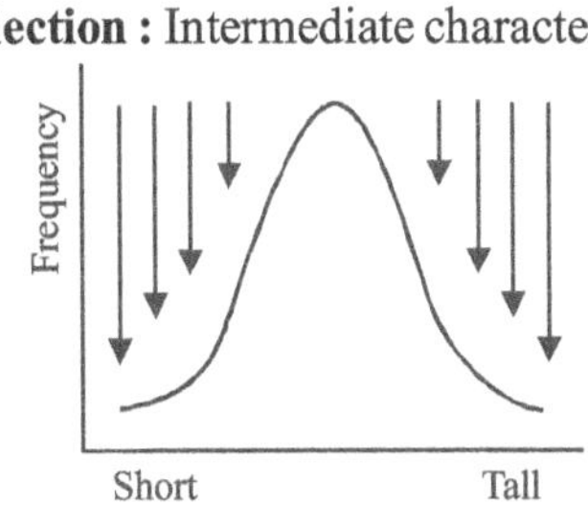

Height variation in humans

  - **Directional selection :** One of the two possible extremes is favoured.

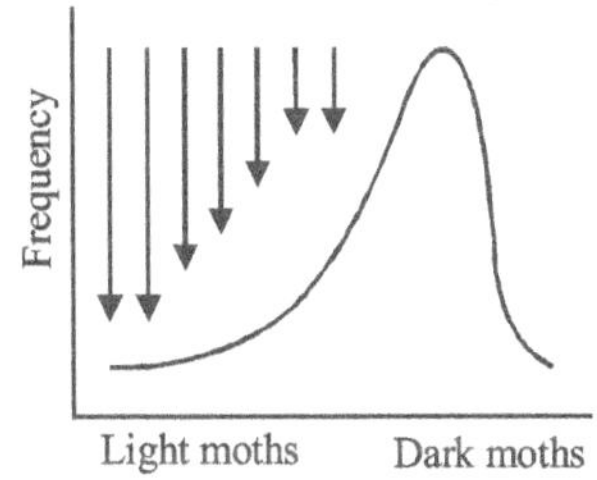

Industrial melanism

– **Disruptive selection :** Natural selection moves characteristics toward both extremes, and intermediate phenotypes become rarest.

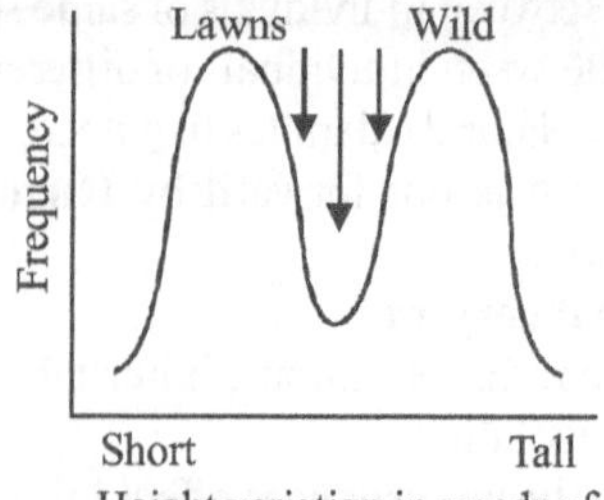

Height variation in weeds of lawns and in the wild

EVIDENCES OF EVOLUTIONS

- **Paleontological evidences** for evolution refer to the evidences from fossils.
- Fossils are the naturally preserved remains or traces of organisms that lived in the geologic past. These organisms are preserved in the form of skeletal, foot prints, trails, casts and moulds, resin (amber) etc. They are **generally found in sedimentary rocks.**
- **Paleontology** is the study of fossils.
- **Geological time scale** is an essential tool for understanding the history of Earth and the evolution of life.
- It indicates the sequence and duration of eras and periods with their dominant forms of life.
- **Divergent evolution and homologous organ :** Whale, bats, cheetah and human (all animals) share similarities in pattern of bones of forelimb. Though they perform different function but they have same anatomical structure. Thus in these animals, same structure developed along different direction for adaptation to different needs. This is **divergent evolution** and structures are **homologous.**
- Homology indicates common ancestory. **Other examples are**
  - Vertebrate hearts or brains
  - Thorn and tendrils of *Bougainvillea* and *Cucurbita.*
- **Analogous organs** are the result of **convergent or parallel evolution** in separate lineage. Different structures evolve for same function and have similarity.
- Analogous organs are not anatomically similar enough though they perform similar functions. E.g.,
  - Wings of butterfly and birds
  - Eyes of octopus and mammals
  - Flippers of penguins and dolphins
  - Sweet potato (root modification) and potato (stem modification)
- **Missing link** is the transitional forms between two groups of organisms occurring only in the fossil state. Eg. *Archaeopteryx*.
- **Vestigial organs** are the useless & functionless degenerate structures which were large and functional in some other animals.
  Examples are vermiform appendix, coccyx, pinna muscle, wisdom tooth in man etc.

- **Adaptive radiation** is a special evolutionary pattern, characterised by a rapid increase in number of kinds of closely related species.
  A **good example of adaptive radiation** is found among the Finches of Galapagos Islands.

ORIGIN AND EVOLUTION OF MAN

- **Paleoanthropology** is the scientific study of human evolution.
- Humans, chimpanzees, gorillas, and the large apes of Africa **share a common ancestor** that lived between eight million and five million years ago.
- Humans, or hominids, belong to the scientific order named Primates (that includes the monkeys, lemurs, and apes) of class mammalia.
- Many experts believe that Australopithecus garhi or a similar species gave rise to the genus *Homo*.
- Early hominids– members of the genus Homo–lived contemporaneously with australopithecines for perhaps a half million years.
- The oldest fossil remains of a member of the genus Homo were discovered in Tanzania. It was named *H. habilis*.
- *Homo erectus* is the **only other known extinct species of the genus Homo**.
- H. erectus was replaced in tropical regions by Homo sapiens about 200,000 years ago.
- Cro-Magnon man used to carry domesticated dogs while going for hunting.
- The most accepted line of descent in human evolution is –
  Ramapithecus → Homo habilis → Homo erectus → Homo sapiens.
  The **first hominid** was known as *Homo habilis*.

EXERCISE

1. **Explain antibiotic resistance observed in bacteria in light of Darwinian selection theory.**

Sol. According to Darwinian selection theory, the organisms with the important characteristic features that enable them to survive better in natural conditions (the existing environmental conditions) would eliminate the others organisms that are less-endowed to survive under those conditions.

An example of such selection is antibiotic resistance in bacteria. Bacteria have been subjected to antibiotics since the earliest discovery of the first antibiotic *i.e.* Penicillin. When these bacterial populations are grown in culture containing antibiotic penicillin, the colonies that were sensitive to penicillin died, whereas one or few bacterial colonies that were resistant to penicillin survived. Only the ones that survived the antibiotic treatment could further perpetuate and produce offsprings, resulting in the increase of antibiotic resistance in the bacterial population.

Hence, the resistant bacteria multiplied quickly as compared to non- resistant (sensitive) bacteria, thereby increasing their number. Hence, the advantage of an individual over other helps in the struggle for existence.

Note

- *According to Darwinian selection theory, bacteria can acquire resistance in two ways: either through a new genetic change that helps the bacterium survives, or by getting DNA from a bacterium that is already resistant.*
- *The use of antibiotics or drugs against eukaryotic organism has resulted in the selection of resistant varieties in much lesser time. There are examples of evolution by anthropogenic action.*

2. Find out from newspapers and popular science articles any new fossil discoveries or controversies about evolution.

Sol.
- *New fossil discovered* : Palaeontologists from Hokkaido University in Japan, in cooperation with palaeontologists from the Perot Museum of Nature and Science in Dallas, Texas, have discovered the first-confirmed occurrence of a lambeosaurine (crested 'duck-billed' dinosaur) from the Arctic - part of the skull of a lambeosaurine dinosaur from the Liscomb Bonebed (71-68 Ma) found on Alaska's North Slope.
  The discovery proves for the first time that lambeosaurines inhabited the Arctic during the Late Cretaceous. In addition, the numeric abundance of hadrosaurine fossils compared to the lambeosaurine fossils in the marine-influenced environment of the Liscomb Bonebed suggests the possibility that hadrosaurines and lambeosaurines had different habitat preferences.
  A fossil of human was discovered in Israel. This fossil has been named as Misliya-1; after the cave in which it was found. Previously scientists believed that Homo sapiens left Africa around 100,000 years ago. But this fossil makes the scientists estimate that Homo sapiens may have left Africa about 175,000 to 200,000 years ago.
- *Controversies about evolution*
  (i) Huxley proposed that man evolved from the apes but paleontological evidences revealed that man and apes had common ancestry.
  (ii) Earlier the spermatophytes were considered to be the first seed-bearing plants but the fossil studies have shown that Pteridosperms (seed ferns) were first land plants to develop seed habit. These act as missing link between the Ferns and Gymnosperms.

Note

- *This new discovery of lambeosaurine (crested 'duck-billed' dinosaur) exemplifies the geographic link between lambeosaurines of North America and the Far East.*
- *Part of a jawbone found in Misliya, Israel, has been identified as the oldest human fossil found outside Africa.*

3. Attempt giving a clear definition of the term species.

Sol. Species is population or group of individuals that have potential of interbreeding in order to produce viable, fertile young ones but are reproductively isolated from members of other species.

4. Try to trace the various components of human evolution (hint: brain size and function, skeletal structure, dietary preference, etc.)

Sol. During human evolution, ancestral human types had undergone a number of remarkable changes in their brain size (cranial capacity), skeletal features/ posture, dietary preference, features etc., as shown in the given table.

S. No.	Stage of human evolution	Component of human evolution			Features
		Brain size and function	Skeletal structures/Posture	Dietary preferences	
1.	*Dryopithecus africans*	—	Knuckle walker, walked similar to gorillas and chimpanzees (was more ape-like).	Herbivorous (Soft fruit and leaves).	Canines large, arms and legs are of equal size.
2.	*Ramapithecus*	—	Semi-erect (more man-like)	Herbivorous (Seeds, nuts)	Canines were small while molars were large.
3.	*Australopithecus africanus*	450 cm^3	Full erect posture, height (1.05 m)	Herbivorous (ate fruits)	Hunted with stone weapons, lived at trees, canines and incisors were small.
4.	*Homo habilis*	650 – 800 cc	Fully erect posture, height (1.5 m)	Carnivorous (feeding on other animals)	Canines were small. They were first tool makers.
5.	*Homo erecius*	900 cc.	Fully erect posture, height(1.5–1.8 m)	Omnivorous (feeding on a variety of food of both plant and animal origin)	They used stone and bone tools for hunting games.

Contd....

6.	*Homo neanderthalnsis*	1400 cc	Fully erect posture, height (1.5–1.66 m)	Omnivorous (feeding on a variety of food of both plant and animal origin).	Cave dwellers, used hides to protect their bodies, and buried their dead.
7.	*Homo sapiens fossilis*	1650 cm^3	Fully erect posture with height (1.8 m)	Omnivorous (feeding on a variety of food of both plant and animal origin).	They had strong jaw with teeth close together. They were cave dwellers, made paintings and carvings in the caves. They developed a culture and were called first modern men.
8.	*Homo sapiens sapiens*	1200–1600 cm^3	Fully erect posture, height (1.5–1.8 m)	Omnivorous (feeding on a variety of food of both plant and animal origin).	They are the living modern men, with high intelligence. They developed art, culture, language, speech, etc. They cultivated crops and domesticated animals.

Note

Don't leave the following topics regarding human evolution.

- *Sequence of origin*
- *Place of fossil discovery*
- *Cranial capacity of brain*

5. **Find out through internet and popular science articles whether animals other than man has self-consciousness.**

Sol. There are many animals other than humans which have self consciousness. Self consciousness may be defined as aware of oneself as an individual. Recent studies on self consciousness says that *dolphin* is *the best example that have self consciousness like man*. Recognising oneself in a mirror is an indicator of self awareness.

Because, dolphins are highly intelligent mammals. They have a sense of self and they also recognize others among themselves and others. They exhibit intimacy and chemistry with their partners and communicate with through various body gestures including whistles, tail-slapping, and other body movements.

Not only dolphins but there are some other animals also such as Chimpanzees, Bottlenose dolphins, Gorillas, Orcas and even elephants which have been observed to show variable levels of self-consciousness. Apes, like the human beings, have well developed facial muscles for showing facial gestures and also have property of self-consciousness.

> ***Note***
>
> *Self-consciousness is the ability to introspect and identify self from the others. It is checked through various techniques and one such is mirror test in which many animals including Dolphins passed.*

6. **List 10 modern-day animals and using the internet resources link it to a corresponding ancient fossil. Name both.**

Sol.

S. No.	Animal	Ancient Fossil	Feature
1.	Dog	Leptocyon	Small extinct genus of canid endemic to North America during the Oligocene through Miocene living from 24.8–10.3 million years ago, existing for about 14.5 million years. It was a small-bodied, fox-like animal with a slender jaw.
2.	Whale	*Protocetus*	An extinct species of primitive cetacean from Egypt. It lived during the middle Eocene period 45 million years ago.
3.	Man	*Ramapithecus*	An extinct group of primates that lived from about 12 to 14 million years ago, for a time regarded as a possible ancestor of Australopithecus and, therefore, of modern humans. Fossils of Ramapithecus were discovered in N India and in E Africa, beginning in 1932.

Contd...

4.	Camel	*Protylopus*	An extinct genus of camel that lived during middle to late Eocene some 45-40 million years ago in North America.
5.	Elephant	Moeritherium	An extinct genus of primitive proboscideans. These prehistoric mammals are related to the elephant and, more distantly, sea cows and hyraxes. They lived during the Eocene epoch.
6.	Bat	*Archaeonycteris*	A primitive bat genus whose remains were found in Germany, France, England and India.
7.	Giraffe	*Palaeotragus* ("*ancient goat*")	A genus of very large, primitive, okapi-like giraffes from the Miocene of Africa and Eurasia.
8.	Horse	*Eohippus*	An extinct genus of small equid ungulates. Eohippus (genus Hyracotherium), also called dawn horse, is an extinct group of mammals that were the first known horses. They flourished in North America and Europe during the early part of the Eocene Epoch (56 million to 33.9 million years ago).
9.	Tetrapoda	Ichthyostega	A Genus of extinct animals whose fossils are found in rocks in eastern Greenland from late Devonian period. It is about one metre long and had a small dorsal fin along the margin of its tail.
10.	Bird	*Archaeopteryx*	A genus of bird-like dinosaurs that is transitional between non-avian feathered dinosaurs and modern birds.

7. Practise drawing various animals and plants.

Sol. You can take help from your book and Internet to draw various animals and plants.

(1) 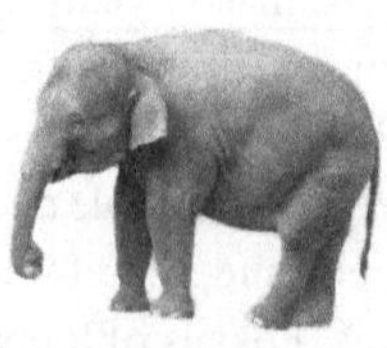

Elephant

(2) 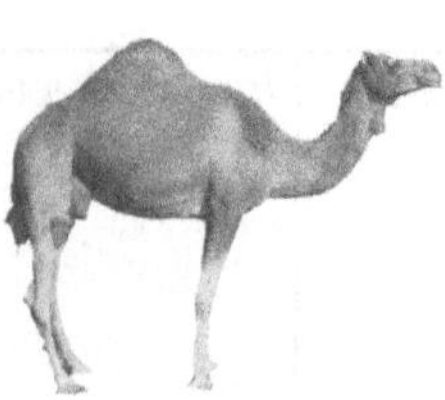

Camel

(3) 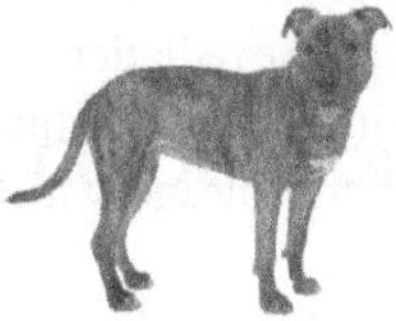 (4) 

Dog **Rose**

(5) 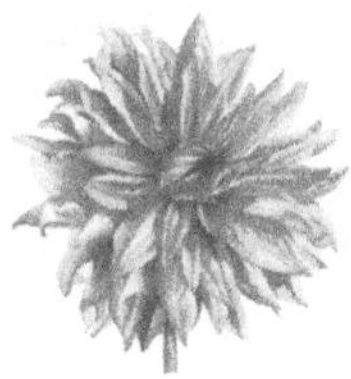 (6) 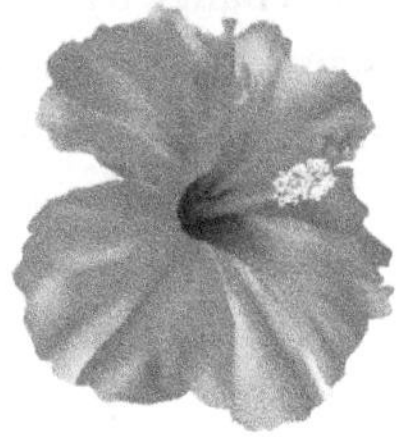

Dahlia **Hibiscus**

8. **Describe one example of adaptive radiation.**

Sol. Adaptive radiation is an evolutionary process that produces new species from a single, rapidly diversifying lineage. This process occurs due to natural selection. An *example of adaptive radiation is Darwin finches*, found in Galapagos Island.

A large variety of finches is present in Galapagos Island that arose from a single species, which reached this land accidentally. As a result, many new species have evolved, diverged, and adapted to occupy new habitats. These finches have developed different eating habits and different types of beaks to suit their feeding habits. The insectivorous, blood sucking, and other species of finches with varied dietary habits have evolved from a single seed eating finch ancestor.

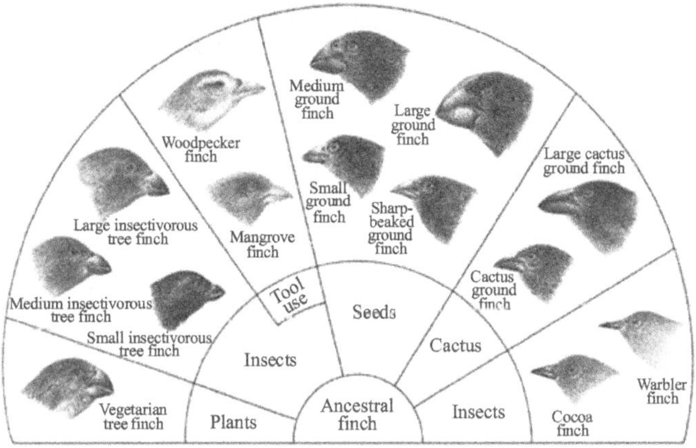

Fig.: Darwin finches of Galapagos Island

Darwin's finches of the Galapagos islands had common ancestors but now have different types of modified beaks according to their food habits.

9. Can we call human evolution as adaptive radiation?

Sol.
- No, we cannot call human evolution as adaptive radiation.
- *Because*, adaptive radiation is an evolutionary process that produces new species from a single, rapidly diversifying lineage, which is not the case with human evolution.

  Human evolution is a gradual process that took place slowly in time. It is a process of change by which people originated from apelike ancestors. It represents an example of anagenesis (= species formation without branching of the evolutionary line of descent).

Homo sapiens sapiens
(25,000 years, 1.5–1.8 M, 1300–1600 c.c.)
↑
Homo sapiens fossils
(34,000 years 1.8 M, 1650 c.c.)
↑
Homo erectus
(1.7 million years, 800–1100 c.c.)
↑
Homo habilis
(2 million years, 735 c.c., First fossil man who used tools of chipped stones)
↑
Australopithecus africanus
(5 million years 1.5 m, 350–450 c.c.)
↑
Ramapithecus
(14–15 million years, survived from Late Miocene to pliocene)
↑
Apes ← *Dryopithecus africanus*
(20–25 million years)

Fig.: Schematic representation of human evolution

Note

- *Hominid introduction occured in Africa and Asia.*
- Homo habilis *lived in Africa – 2 million years ago.*
- Homo erectus– *migrated to Asia and Europe and diverged into 2 species – Java Man and Peking Man.*
- *Similarly* Homo erectus – *was followed by* Homo sapiens.
- *Primitive neanderthal man in Europe gave way to African cro-magnon.*

10. Using various resources such as your school library or the internet and discussions with your teacher, trace the evolutionary stages of any one animal say horse.

Sol.
- The evolution of horse started with Eohippus during Eocene period. It involved the following evolutionary changes:
  - (i) Gradual increase in body size.
  - (ii) Elongation of head and neck region.
  - (iii) Increase in the length of limbs and feet.
  - (iv) Gradual reduction of lateral digits.
  - (v) Enlargement of third functional toe.
  - (vi) Strengthening of the back.
  - (vii) Development of brain and sensory organs.
  - (viii) Increase in the complexity of teeth for feeding on grass.
- The *evolutionary stages of horse* is represented as follow:
  - (i) *Hyracotherium or Eohippus*: They are also called dawn horse. Evolution of horse started with eohippus. It had a short head and neck and four functional toes with a splint of 1 and 5 on each hind limb and a splint of 1 and 3 in each forelimb. The molars were short crowned that were adapted for grinding the plant diet.
  - (ii) *Mesohippus (Intermediate horse)*: It was slightly taller than Eohippus. It had three toes in each foot. Fossil of mesohippus are found in the early and middle oligocene of North America. It also had a larger brain.
  - (iii) *Merychippus*: It had the size of approximately 100 cm. Although it still had three toes in each foot, but it could run on one toe. The side toe did not touch the ground. The molars were adapted for chewing the grass.
  - (iv) *Pliohippus*: It resembled the modern horse and was around 108 cm tall. It had a single functional toe with splint of 2nd and 4th in each limb.
  - (v) *Equus*: Pliohippus gave rise to Equus or the modern horse with one toe in each foot. They have incisors for cutting grass and molars for grinding food. This horse was about the size of a fox terrier.

Note

Horse fossils have been found in sedimentary strata at the beginning of the Tertiary period during a time-span called the Eocene (approximately 50 million years ago, according to uniformitarian dating). They are usually labelled Eohippus or Hyracotherium.

Chapter 8

HUMAN HEALTH AND DISEASE

CHAPTER AT A GLANCE

- **Health** is a state of complete physical, social and mental well being and not merely the absence of disease or infirmity.
- **Disease** is any condition which interferes with the normal structure & function of the body that is manifested by a characteristics sets of symptoms & sign.
- **Infection** is the process by which harmful microorganism enters the body and makes them ill or diseases.
- **Contamination** refers to the presence of disease-causing agents in nonliving things like water, food etc.
- **Infestation** is the presence of an unusually large number of insects or animals in a place, typically so as to cause damage or disease.
- Diseases are of **two types on the basis of their occurrence**: congenital and acquired. **Congenital diseases** are inborn diseases whereas **acquired disease** occurs only after birth. They are further of two types: communicable and non-communicable.
- **Communicable (infectious) diseases** are caused by viruses, rickettsia, bacteria, fungi, protozoans and worms and **non-communicable (non-infectious) diseases** remain confined to the person who develops them and do not spread to others.
- **Disease caused by bacteria** are typhoid, pneumonia, dysentery, plague, diphtheria, etc.
- **Typhoid** is caused by bacterium *Salmonella typhi*. Symptoms are high fever, headache, weakness, loss of apetite, skin rash, constipation, stomach ache etc. Typhoid is **diagnosed with widal test**.
- **Pneumonia** is an infection of lung which is caused by bacteria, virus, fungi or parasites. It is a type of chest infection which affects the tiny air sacs (called alveoli) in your lungs. In this condition these air sacs get inflamed and fill with fluid which makes it harder to breathe. It is characterised by difficulty in respiration, fever, chills, cough, and headache. It is caused by bacteria like *Streptococcus pneumoniae* and *Haemophilus influenza*.
- **Diseases caused by virus** are common cold, small pox, measles, mumps, poliomyelitis, dengue, yellow fever, rabies etc.
- Rhinoviruses causes one of the most infectious disease called **common cold.** Droplets resulting from cough or sneezes of an infected person are either inhaled directly or transmitted through contaminated objects.

- **Diseases caused by protozoans** are malaria, amoebiasis, giardiasis, Kala azar, trypanosomiasis etc.
- **Malaria**
  - Malaria is caused by *Plasmodium* species & spread through female *Anopheles* mosquito. Primary host are female mosquito of genus *Anopheles* & humans acts as intermediate host.
  - *Plasmodium* enters the human body as sporozoites (**infectious form**) through the bite of infected female *Anopheles* mosquito.
- **Amoebic dysentery or amoebiasis**
  - It is caused by *Entamoeba histolytica.*
  - It is transmitted by poor sanitation and contamination of drinking water or food by faeces of infected persons. Houseflies acts as mechanical carriers & serve to transmit the parasite from faeces of infected person to food & its products thereby contaminating them.
- **Filariasis** is caused by *Wuchereria bancrofti*. It is also known as **elephantiasis** due to excessive enlargement of body parts like legs.
- **Ascariasis**
  - It is caused by *Ascaris lumbricoides* and it is more common in children.
  - Vectors for ascariasis are flies or cockroaches containing embryonated eggs of *Ascaris* contaminated with food & water.
  - Ascariasis is characterised by colic pain, fever, indigestion, diarrhoea, vomiting, weakness, retarded physical & mental efficiency, internal bleeding, muscular pain, blockage of intestinal passage.
- **Fungi causes diseases** and these are known as **mycosis**. *Microsporum, Trichophyton* and *Epidermophyton* are responsible for **ringworms**, which is characterised by appearance of dry scaly lesions of the skin, nails and scalps.

CANCER

- Cancer is a disease caused by an uncontrolled division of abnormal cells in a part of the body.
- Cancer can sometimes spread to other parts of the body - this is called a secondary tumour or a **metastasis**.
- Cancer and its treatments can affect body systems, such as the blood circulation, lymphatic and immune systems, and the hormone system.
- Tumours are usually divided into benign and malignant. A **benign tumour** is localised, develops slowly and does not usually result in the patient's death. **Malignant or cancerous tumours** develop more rapidly. They are not localised and are often fatal for the patient.
- **Carcinogens** are factors or physical or chemical agents which induces the cancer growth. *E.g.* coal tar, asbestos, cadmium oxides, etc.
- Cancer causing viruses are called **oncogenic virus**. They have genes called viral oncogenes. In contrast, several genes called proto-onco genes or cellular oncogenes (c-onc) have been identified in normal cells which, when activated under certain conditions, could lead to oncogenic transformations of the cells.

AIDS

- **AIDS (Acquired Immuno Deficiency Syndrome)** is a chronic life threatening disorder which damages the human body's immune system.
- It is caused by Human Immuno Deficiency Virus (HIV) which is retrovirus having envelope enclosing the RNA genome.
- The major cell affected by HIV is the helper T-lymphocytes.
- The HIV multiplies & slowly begins to destroy the CD_4 lymphocytes (T cells or helper cells) a type of white blood cells (WBC) which is responsible for the coordination of the entire immune system.
- AIDS occurs when **CD_4 cell count falls below 200 cells/mm^3** and vulnerable to opportunistic infections.
- AIDS is diagnosed by **ELISA (Enzyme Linked Immuno Sorbent Assay)**. Commonly used enzyme is ELISA techniques are **peroxidases** and **alkaline phosphate**.
- The medicine used to treat HIV is called antiviral therapy or ART.

IMMUNE SYSTEM

- The system of human body which protects it from various infectious agents & cancer is known as **immune system**.
- Immunity against infectious disease is of two types : innate immunity and acquired immunity.
- **Innate immunity** is developed in an individual without having the disease or immunisation, e.g., recreation of sweat glands contain certain chemical substances which prevent the entry of micro-organisms. It is also called **non-specific defence mechanism**. It is present from birth.
- The resistance against infectious disease that an individual acquires during life is known as **acquired immunity.**
- Acquired immunity occurs after exposure to an agent, is specific and is mediated by antibody and T lymphocyte (T cells, cytotoxic cells).
- Active acquired immunity may be **natural** or **artificial**.
- In **natural active acquired immunity**, antibody production is stimulated by living organisms or their products which cause the disease.
- The resistance that is transmitted to recipient in a ready-made form is known as **passive acquired immunity**. There is no antigenic stimulus. There is no active role of immune system of the recipient. The immunity is transient, lasting for a few days or weeks.
- **Immunoglobulin** is blood proteins, produced by plasma cells as an immune response against foreign agents (antigens).
- Inoculation of vaccines to prevent diseases is called **immunisation**.
- **Vaccines** are preparations of living or killed micro-organisms or their products. Vaccines are of two types – live vaccines and killed vaccines.
- **Genetic vaccines** involve one or more genes from diseases carrying agent (pathogen) and splicing these gene into plasmids (closed rings of DNA).
- **Allergy** is a hypersensitivity reaction acquired through exposure to a particular allergens that can involves various deleterious effects such as Hay fever, asthma, serum sickness, systemic anaphylaxis.

DRUG AND ALCOHOL ABUSE

- Drugs are classified on the basis of mode of action on brain into 2 categories:
  - **Psychotropic or psychoactive drugs** (mood altering or neurological drugs).
  - **Psychedelic or hallucinogenic drugs.**
- Commonly abused drugs are **opioids, cannabinoids** and **coca, alkaloids.**
- **Nicotine acts as tranquilisers** but also stimulates the release of adrenaline leading to high blood pressure.
- **Adolescence** is the period of rapid growth, the physical & mental development poised between childhood & adulthood (between 8-18 years for girls and 7-19 years of boys).
- **Addiction** refers to the dependence on and craving for tobacco, alcohol or a particular drug.
- **Alcoholism** is the consumption of or pre-ccupation with alcoholic beverages to the extent that this behavour interferes with the alcoholic's normal personal, family life.
- Alcohol decreases the activity of CNS thereby reducing anxiety, tensions & inhibitions. It also decreases the ADH secretion causing increased urine output.
- Excessive doses of drugs may lead to coma & death due to respiratory, heart failure & cerebral haemorrhage.

EXERCISE

1. What are the various public health measures, which you would suggest as safeguard against infectious diseases?

Sol. Public health measures are preventive measures which are taken to check the spread of various infectious diseases. These measures should be taken to reduce the contact with infectious agents. Minimising- the transmission of infectious disease is a core function of public health law.

The *various public health measures against infectious diseases* includes the following –

(i) *Education* – People should be educated about the infectious diseases so that they may protect themselves against the infections.

(ii) *Isolation* – A people suffering from any infections should be isolated to avoid its transmission to any other person. Isolation can reduce the chances of spreading of airborne diseases such as pneumonia, chicken pox, tuberculosis etc.

(iii) *Sanitation* – Sanitary surroundings can prevent spread of diseases. Maintenance of personal and public hygiene is one of the most important methods of preventing infectious diseases. Public hygiene includes – suitable disposal of waste & human excreta; periodic cleaning and disinfection of water sources; observing normal practices of hygiene in public catering. Personal hygiene includes keeping the body clean, intake of clean drinking water, consumption of healthy and nutritious food, vegetables, fruits etc.

(iv) *Vaccination* – It is the protection of the body against communicable diseases. It is a process of injecting killed microbe in order to stimulate the immune system against the microbe, thereby preventing disease. It helps in providing passive immunisation to the body. Several vaccines are available against many diseases like tetanus, polio, measles, mumps, etc.

(v) *Vector eradication* – Vector is an organism that transmits a disease or parasite from one animal to another. It is a carrier of several diseases like malaria, filariasis, dengue, and chikungunya etc. These diseases can be prevented by providing a clean environment and by preventing the breeding of mosquitoes. This can be achieved by not allowing water to stagnate around residential areas.

Also, measures like regular cleaning of coolers, use of mosquito nets and insecticides (such as Malathion) in drains, ponds, etc. can be undertaken to ensure a healthy environment. Introducing laxvivorous fish such as *Gambusia* in ponds also controls the breeding of mosquito larvae in stagnant water.

2. In which way has the study of biology helped us to control infectious diseases?

Sol. Infectious diseases are disorders caused by pathogenic organisms, such as bacteria, viruses, fungi or parasites. Many organisms which live in and on our bodies, are normally harmless or even helpful, but under certain conditions, some organisms may cause disease.

These infectious diseases can be spread through various means, like

- From person to person.
- By bites from insects or animals.
- By ingesting contaminated food or water or being exposed to organisms in the environment.

Each infectious disease has its own specific signs and symptoms. General signs and symptoms common to a number of infectious diseases include: fever, diarrhoea, fatigue, muscle aches, coughing etc.

The *study of biology helped us to control these infectious diseases* because a particular branch of biological science (called pathology) helps us to study the causes and effects of disease by examining the samples of body tissue. These examination can be done for diagnostic or forensic purposes:

Advancements achieved in biological science also helped us gain a better understanding to fight against various infectious diseases and to understand various aspects of life, like the shape, structure and function of living organisms, the evolution of life, etc.

Methods of biological science to control infectious diseases can be done by studying the following:

(i) *Life cycle of parasites, etc*: With respect to human health, it helped us study the life cycle of various parasites, pathogens, and vectors along with its modes of transmission and the measures for controlling them.

(ii) *Vaccine*: Discovery of vaccines and their timely use in immunisation programmes have helped in controlling and even eradicating certain infectious diseases. These programmes against several infectious diseases such as small pox, chicken pox, tuberculosis, etc. have helped eradicate these diseases.

(iii) *Drugs and antibiotics*: Biotechnology has also helped in the preparation of newer and safer drugs and vaccines to cure disorders. Discovery of antibiotics and other drugs have also played an important role in treating infectious diseases.

3. How does the transmission of each of the following diseases take place?
(a) Amoebiasis (b) Malaria (c) Ascariasis (d) Pneumonia

Sol. (a) Amoebiasis

- It is a disease caused by the parasite *Entamoeba histolytica*.
- *Mode of transmission*
  (i) It is transmitted by the faecal-oral route.
  (ii) It is also transmitted indirectly through contact with dirty hands or objects.
  (iii) Through ingestion of the cyst form (called amoebic cyst) of the parasite, a semi-dormant and hardy structure found in faeces.
  (iv) The vector involved in the transmission is housefly.

(b) Malaria

- It is a life-threatening mosquito-borne blood protozoan disease, caused by *Plasmodium* species.
- *Mode of transmission*
  (i) Bite by an infected female mosquito of the genus *Anopheles*, which previously had stung a person infected with malaria.
  (ii) The mosquito picks up the parasite along with the blood when it bites an infected person. When this mosquito bites an other healthy person, the parasites migrate into his blood with the saliva, which the mosquito injects before sucking up blood to prevent its clotting.

Note

Less common ways of transmission of malaria are: blood transfusion, transplantation, infected needles, from mother to foetus during pregnancy.

(c) Ascariasis

- It is a roundworm infection, caused by *Ascaris lumbricoides*.
- *Mode of transmission* : Through contaminated soil mixed with human faeces that contain ascariasis eggs or infected water.

(d) Pneumonia

- A variety of organisms, including bacteria, viruses and fungi, can cause pneumonia. The most common are bacteria and viruses in the air we breathe. The most common cause of bacterial pneumonia is *Streptococcus pneumoniae*. *Haemophilus influenzae* type b (Hib) - the second most common cause of bacterial pneumonia. *Mycoplasma pneumoniae* also can cause pneumonia.
- *Mode of transmission*
  (i) The viruses and bacteria that are commonly found in a child's nose or throat can infect the lungs if they are inhaled.

(ii) They may also spread via air-borne droplets from a cough or sneeze.

(iii) In addition, pneumonia may spread through blood, especially during and shortly after birth.

4. What measures would you take to prevent water-borne diseases?

Sol.
- Water-borne diseases are any disease caused by drinking water contaminated by human or animal faeces, which contain pathogenic microorganisms.
- Examples of water borne diseases are cholera, typhoid, hepatitis B, etc.
- *Water borne diseases can be prevented* by the following:

(i) Oral Rehydration Solution (ORS) : It is used to prevent dehydration and electrolyte loss. It is a special combination of dry salts that is mixed with safe water. It can help reduce the fluids lost due to diarrhoea.

(ii) Health education

(iii) General hygiene, pure water : Water bodies, ponds, water tank reservoirs in the city or village should be cleaned periodically.

(iv) Vaccination and immunisation : Vaccination is an effective method to control the outcome of water-borne diseases. For example, two oral cholera vaccines that were used in mass vaccination campaigns. Today, they are considered an effective tool against high-risk cholera and are being implemented worldwide.

(v) By ensuring proper disposal of sewage excreta, periodic cleaning.

(vi) Do not drink untreated water from a spring, river, stream, lake, pond etc.

(vii) Personal hygiene : A personal level, practice good hygiene such as frequent hand washing and disinfection of cutlery, cutting boards, etc. Wash hands thoroughly and frequently using soap, in particular after contact with pets or farm animals, or after having been to the toilet.

Note

Water-borne disease is easily transmitted when contaminated water is used for any of the following purposes: drinking, making ice cubes, washing uncooked fruits and vegetables, making baby formula, brushing teeth and washing dentures or contact lenses.

5. Discuss with your teacher what does 'a suitable gene' means, in the context of DNA vaccines.

Sol. DNA vaccines are third generation vaccines. They are made up of small, circular pieces of bacterial DNA, plasmids which are genetically engineered to produce specific antigens from a pathogen. After administration of the DNA, antigens are produced and stimulate an immune response.

Similarly, a *suitable gene* in the context of DNA vaccines is the specific segment of DNA which injected into the host in the form of vaccine. This segment has the ability to produce specific proteins.

This gene which encode a protein associated with the target infectious organism, is spliced into plasmid, then copied & formulated as a vaccine. This protein act as an antigen, kills the specific disease-causing organism in the host body and provides immunity against the disease.

6. Name the primary and secondary lymphoid organs.

Sol. Lymphoid organs are those organs of immune system, in which lymphocytes can differentiate and proliferate. They are part of the lymphatic system which defend the body against invading pathogens that cause infections or spread of tumours. These organs exist as primary, secondary or tertiary based on the stage of lymphocyte development and maturation the organ is involved in.

- The *primary lymphoid organs consist* of specialised tissue, in which generation and maturation of B- and T-lymphocytes takes place. Primary lymphoid organs are *bone marrow and thymus*. Both bone marrow and thymus provide micro-environments for the development and maturation of T-lymphocytes.
- *Secondary lymphoid organs* provide the sites for the interaction of lymphocytes with the antigen, which then proliferate to become effector cells. Secondary lymphoid organs are *spleen* (white pulp of spleen), *lymph nodes* and *MALT* (tonsils, Peyer's patches of small intestine and appendix).

> ***Note***
>
> *Tertiary lymphoid organs usually contains less number of lymphocytes. It plays an important role during inflammation. Inflammation protects the body by removing harmful stimuli and initiating a healing process.*

7. The following are some well-known abbreviations, which have been used in this chapter. Expand each one to its full form:

(a) MALT (b) CMI (c) AIDS (d) NACO (e) HIV

Sol.

	Abbreviations	Expanded form	Description
(a)	MALT	Mucosal-Associated Lymphoid Tissue	• It constitutes the most extensive component of human lymphoid tissue and scattered along mucosal linings in the human body. • Examples: tonsils, the Peyer's patches within the small intestine, and the appendix. • It allows immune system to sample microbial antigens for development of adaptive immune responses and provides a location for plasma cells to synthesise IgA.

Contd....

(b)	CMI	Cell-Mediated Immunity	• It refers to protective mechanisms that are not primarily characterised by antibody. • It is responsible for detecting and destroying intracellular pathogens. • It is important for graft rejection and destruction of tumor cells and for delayed-type hypersensitivity reactions.
(c)	AIDS	Acquired Immune Deficiency Syndrome	• It is the final or advance stage of HIV (human deficiency syndrome) infection. • It alters the immune system, making people more vulnerable to infections and diseases. • It spreads through unprotected sex with an infected person, sharing drug needles or through contact with the blood of an infected person.
(d)	NACO	National AIDS Control Organisation	• It is a division of the Ministry of Health and Family Welfare, Government of India. • It was established in 1992 with the aim of providing leadership to the HIV/AIDS control Programme in India. • It is headquartered at New Delhi.
(e)	HIV	Human Immune Deficiency virus	• It is retrovirus which causes AIDS. • It infects and destroys certain white blood cells called CD4+ cells.

8. Differentiate the following and give examples of each.

(a) Innate and acquired immunity

(b) Active and passive immunity

Sol. (a) Difference between innate and acquired immunity

S. No.	Innate immunity	Adaptive/Acquired immunity
1.	It is an inborn resistance against infections that an individual possesses right from the birth, due to his genetic or constitutional mark-up.	It is the resistance against infecting foreign substance that an individual acquires or adapts during the course of life.

Contd....

2.	It is present before the first exposure to microbial antigen. Prior exposure to the antigen is not required, hence considered as first line of defence against pathogen.	It develops during lifetime following the antigenic exposure, hence considered as second line of defence against pathogen.
3.	Components of innate immunity are: anatomical /physiological barrier (like skin, mucous membrane, temperature, pH, chemicals cells, phagocytes (monocytes, macrophages, and neutrophils), natural killer cells, normal resident flora etc.	Components of acquired immunity are T cell, B cell, classical, complement pathway, antigen presenting cells (APC), cytokines etc.
4.	It is non-specific, defends against any pathogen up on first exposure.	It is antigen specific and responds to specific pathogen on 2nd or latter exposure.
5.	Does not produce allergic reactions.	Develops allergic reactions, immediate and delayed hypersensitivity.
6.	Immune response occurs in minutes. It has a limited and lower potency.	It takes days to generate immune response. It has highly potent immune response.
7.	It develops against antigens that are shared by many microbes (called pathogens-associated molecular patterns).	Acquired immunity develops against antigens that are specific for each microbe.
8.	Immunological memory is absent. It reacts with equal potency upon repeated exposure to same pathogen.	Immunological memory is present. Presence of memory cells triggers a faster and potent response when re-exposed to same pathogens.
9.	It is inheritable.	It is heritable from mother to neonates for a brief period after birth.
10.	E.g, redness and swelling caused by the white blood cells around a wound.	E.g, vaccination against a virus.

(b) Difference between active and passive immunity

S.No.	Active immunity	Passive immunity
1.	It is a type of acquired immunity in which the body produces its own antibodies against disease-causing antigens.	It is a type of acquired immunity in which readymade antibodies are transferred from one individual to another.
2.	It has a long-lasting effect.	It does not have long lasting effect.
3.	It is slow. It takes time in producing antibodies and giving responses.	It is fast. It provides immediate relief.
4.	Example: Injecting microbes through vaccination inside the body. An allergic reaction is an extreme response to an antigen, resulting from active immunity.	Example: Transfer of antibodies present in the mother's milk to the infant. An example of artificial passive immunity is getting an injection of antisera, which is a suspension of antibody particles. Another example is the injection of snake antivenom following a bite.

9. Draw a well-labelled diagram of an antibody molecule.

Sol. Antibodies are the globular protein belonging to immunoglobulin (Ig) family. This structure consists of two identical light (L) chain polypeptide of about 22000 Da and two identical heavy (H) chain of larger polypeptide of about 55000 Da or more. Hence, an antibody is represented as H_2L_2.
Each light chain is bound to a heavy chain by a disulphide bond and by non-covalent interactions such as salt bride, hydrogen bonds and hydrophobic interaction to form a heterodimer (H-L). Similar non-covalent interaction and disulphide linkage link the two identical heterodimer (H-L) to each other to from basic structure of antibody i.e. dimer of dimer.

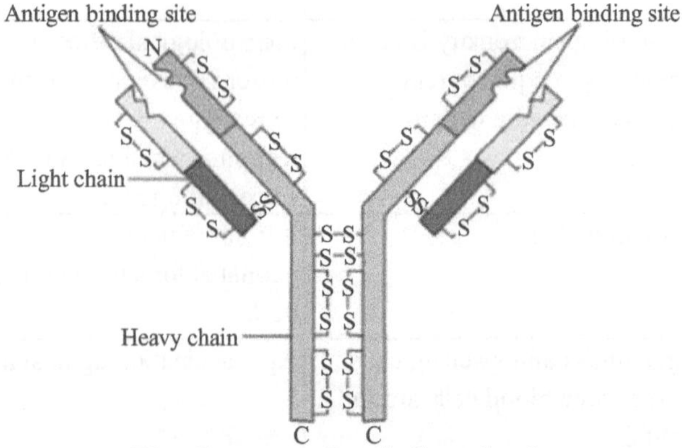

Fig.: Structure of antibody molecule

Note

There are five classes of immunoglobulin-IgA, IgD, IgE, IgG, and IgM-defined by the amino acid sequence of the heavy chain. They have different roles in immune responses; IgG, IgA, and IgM are commonly produced after viral infection.

10. What are the various routes by which transmission of human immunodeficiency virus takes place?

Sol. HIV (Human immunodeficiency virus) is a virus that targets and alters the immune system by attacking immune cells called CD_4 cells, which are a type of T cell, thereby increasing the risk and impact of other infections and diseases. Without treatment, the infection might progress to an advanced disease stage called AIDS (Acquired Immune Deficiency Syndrome). AIDS, the most advanced stage of HIV infection, describes a set of symptoms and illnesses that happen at the final stage of HIV infection, if left untreated. HIV is found in semen, blood, vaginal and anal fluids, and breastmilk. HIV can't be transmitted through sweat, saliva or urine.

Various routes by which transmission of human immuno-deficiency virus takes place are:

(i) Illicit (unprotected or illegal) sexual contact.
(ii) Sexual contact with multiple partners.
(iii) Transfusion of the blood of infected person.
(iv) Intravenous drug users that shares needles are at high risk of contracting AIDS.
(v) From an infected mother to a child through the placenta.

Note

Mosquito can't transmit HIV *because, unlike mosquito borne diseases, HIV is unable to replicate within the mosquito's gut and therefore is broken down. In humans, HIV binds to T cells and begins replicating. No T cells exist inside the mosquito's gut and so the virus has no way of replicating or migrating to the mosquito's salivary glands. HIV particles are therefore digested by the mosquito alongside the actual blood meal. During the digestion process, the HIV particles are "completely destroyed."*

11. What is the mechanism by which the AIDS virus causes deficiency of immune system of the infected person?

Sol. AIDS (Acquired Immune Deficiency Syndrome) is caused by the Human immunodeficiency virus (HIV). The HIV virus enters the human body by various methods like sharing infected needles, unprotected sexual contact with infected person, or infected blood transfusion. HIV critically injures the immune system by infecting and eventually killing T-cells (CD_4 T-cells). As the CD_4 T-cell counts wane, the body becomes progressively more susceptible to opportunistic infection with intracellular microbes.

- *Mechanism by which the AIDS virus causes deficiency of immune system*
  (i) After entering the human body, the HIV virus attacks and enters the macrophages. Inside the macrophages, the RNA of the virus replicates with the help of enzyme reverse transcriptase and gives rise to viral DNA.
  (ii) This process is called reverse transcriptase because it violates the usual way in which genetic information is transcribed. Because reverse transcriptase lacks the proofreading function that most DNA synthesising enzymes have.
  (iii) Then, this viral DNA incorporates into the host DNA and directs the synthesis of virus particles. At the same time, HIV enters helper T-lymphocytes where it replicates and produces viral progeny. These newly formed progeny viruses get released into the blood, attacking other healthy helper T-lymphocytes in the body. As a result, the number of T-lymphocytes in the body of an infected person decreases progressively, thereby decreasing the immunity of a person.
  (iv) Death ultimately results from the relentless attack of opportunistic pathogens or from the body's inability to fight off malignancies.

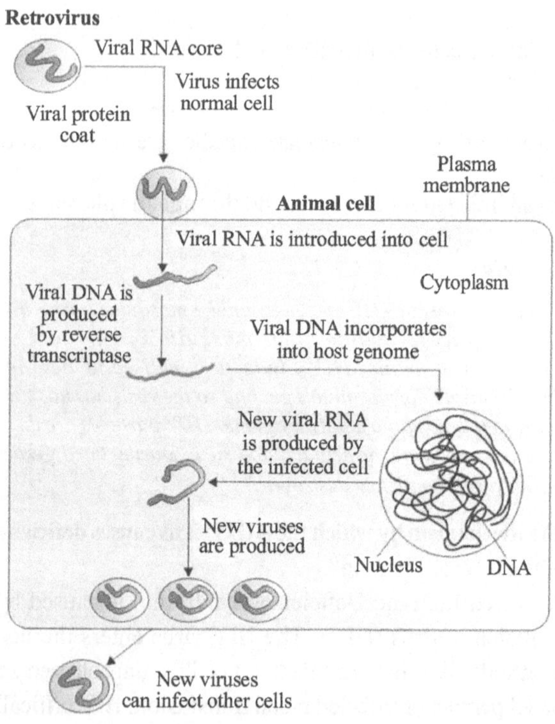

Note

Infected cell can survive while viruses are being replicated and released.

12. How is a cancerous cell different from a normal cell?

Sol. The main difference between cancer cells and normal cells is that the cancer cells have an uncontrolled growth and cell division whereas the growth and cell division of normal cells is controlled.

Difference between cancerous cells from normal cells is given below:

S. No.	Cancer cells	Normal cells
1.	These cells divide relentlessly, forming solid tumours or flooding the blood with abnormal cells.	These are regular body cells that perform a specific function.
2.	It show uncontrolled growth and cell division.	Growth and cell division are controlled.
3.	These cells have a rapid cell division and they divide before their maturation.	These cells stop cell division when the adequate number of cells are present and then undergo maturation.
4.	Do not communicate with nearby cells.	Communicate with nearby cells for homeostatic purposes.
5.	Have altered size and shape.	Have a defined size and shape
6.	Nucleus is larger and darker.	Nucleus is comparatively small and light in colour.
7.	An abnormal number of chromosomes and arrangement.	A defined number of well-arranged chromosomes.
8.	A cluster of cells without a boundary.	Have defined arrangements and boundary.
9.	These cells undergo continuous angiogenesis, which promotes the continuous growth and cell division.	These cells undergo angiogenesis only during the formation of new tissue.
10.	Derive their energy mainly from glycolysis.	20% of the energy comes from glycolysis and 70% comes from the Kreb's cycle.
11.	Not repaired and do not undergo apoptosis.	Repaired and undergo apoptosis when damaged.
12.	These cells have the ability to spread. These cells lack the adhesion molecules that causes stickiness, due to which they are able to travel *via* the blood stream and lymphatic system to the other region of the body.	These cells do not spread (or metastasise) for eg, lung cells remain in the lungs.
13.	Can escape from the detection by the immune system.	Identified and removed by the immune system when damaged.
14.	Do not have a defined function.	Have a defined function.

Note

- *Cancer cells do not have a regular life span.*
- *Not all tumours are cancerous.*

13. Explain what is meant by metastasis.

Sol. Metastasis is a pathological process of spreading cancerous cells from their primary location (the organ in which the cancer began) to the different parts of the body. The property of metastasis is exhibited by malignant tumours. These metastatic cells divide uncontrollably, forming a mass of cells called tumour. From the tumour, some cells get sloughed off and enter into the blood stream. From blood stream these cells reach distant parts of the body and therefore, initiate the formation of new tumours by dividing actively.

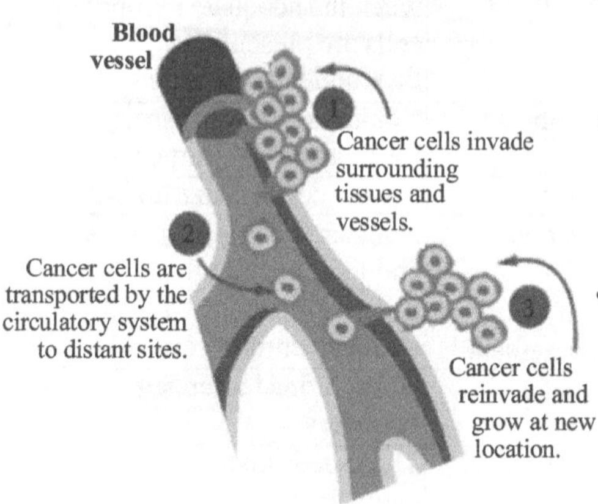

- Abnormal cells proliferate and spread (metastasise) to other parts of the body
- **Invasion - direct migration and penetration into neighbouring tissues**
- **Metastasis - cancer cells penetrate into lymphatic system and blood vessels**

Fig. : Process of metastasis

Note

Cancers can metastasise to nearly any regions of the body, but some of the common sites are the bones, lungs, liver, and brain.

14. List the harmful effects caused by alcohol/drug abuse.

Sol. Alcohol and drugs have several adverse effects on the individual, his family and the society.

- *Harmful effects caused by alcohol abuse*
  (i) Alcohol generates more energy mostly in the form of heat, but at the same time, it dilates the blood vessels. Consequently the heat generated is rapidly lost. Due to constant dilation, the arterial walls soon become brittle & rigid. Such a change in the property of blood vessels & deposition of alcoholic fat affect the working of heart.
  (ii) Alcoholism leads to gastric ulcers & gastritis.
  (iii) In chronic alcoholism, the axon of the nerve inflame thus causing neuritis.

(iv) Permanent damage to liver cells occur due to deposition of fats. The liver dries up & harden (cirrhosis).

(v) Consumption of excess alcohol by any family member can have devastating effects on the family. It leads to several domestic problems such as quarrels, frustrations, insecurity, etc.

- *Harmful effects caused by drug abuse*

(i) Excessive doses of drugs may lead to coma & death due to respiratory failure, heart failure & cerebral haemorrhage.

(ii) It will lead to lack of interest in personal hygiene, withdrawal, isolation, depression, fatigue aggressive & rebellious behaviour etc.

(iii) Acquire serious infections like AIDS & hepatitis B, who take drugs intravenously.

(iv) The adverse effects of drugs are manifested in the form of reckless behaviour, vandalism & violence.

15. Do you think that friends can influence one to take alcohol/drugs? If yes, how may one protect himself/herself from such an influence?

Sol.
- Yes, friends can influence one to take drugs and alcohols.
- A person can take the *following steps for protecting himself/herself against drug abuse*:

(i) Increase your will power to stay away from alcohol and drugs. One should not experiment with alcohol for curiosity and fun.

(ii) Avoid the company of friends who are addicted to drugs and alcohol.

(iii) Seek help from parents and peers.

(iv) Take proper knowledge and counseling about drug abuse.

(v) Devote your energy in other extra-curricular activities.

(vi) Not take undue pressure of failures beyond its threshold.

(vii) Seek immediate professional and medical help from psychologists and psychiatrists if symptoms of depression and frustration become apparent.

16. Why is that once a person starts taking alcohol or drugs, it is difficult to get rid of this habit? Discuss it with your teacher.

Sol. Drug and alcohol consumption has an inherent addictive nature associated with euphoria and a temporary feeling of well-being. Repeated intake of drugs increases the tolerance level of the body's receptors, leading to more consumption of drugs. Psychological & physiological dependence of an individual to the intake of certain kinds of drugs and alcohol is called addiction.

Once a person start taking alcohol & drugs, *it is very difficult to get rid this habit because of the following reasons*:

(i) People with addiction lose control over their actions. They crave and seek out drugs, alcohol, or other substances no matter what the cost-even at the risk of damaging friendships, hurting family, or losing jobs.

(ii) Addiction drive people to take them even when these are not needed or even when their use becomes self destructive.

(iii) With repeated use of drugs, the tolerance level of the receptors present in the body increases, consequently the receptors responds only to higher doses of drugs or alcohol leading to greater intake & addiction. Thus, the addiction potential of drugs & alcohol, pull the user into a vicious circle leading to their regular use (abuse) from which he/she may not able to get out.

Note

Addiction is a disease that affects the brain, but that doesn't mean anyone is helpless. The brain changes associated with addiction can be treated and reversed through therapy, medication, exercise, and other treatments.

17. In your view what motivates youngsters to take to alcohol or drugs and how can this be avoided?

Sol.
- *Factors which motivates youngsters to take alcohol or drugs* : Many factors are responsible for motivating youngsters towards alcohol or drugs, like modern society, curiosity, need for adventure and excitement, experimentation.
  (i) Several mediums like television, internet, newspaper, movies etc. are also responsible for promoting the idea of alcohol to the younger generation. Amongst these factors, reasons such as unstable and unsupportive family structures and peer pressure can also lead an individual to be dependent on drugs and alcohol.
  (ii) Human have probably been using mind – affecting drugs since time immemorial. The root cause of addiction of man to drugs, smoking and drinking has been due to his inability to make mental adjustments with stresses and strains, drudgery and extreme misery in daily life. As a temporary measure, to combat these adverse situations and to have a certain degree of mental relaxation, humans have been making an extensive use of stimulants, depressants and hallucinogens. Stimulants generally speed up body process, and depressants slow them. Hallucinogens can alter a person's thoughts, feelings, and perception.
- *Preventive measures against addiction of alcohol and drugs*
  (i) Parents should motivate and try to increase the will power of their child.
  (ii) Parents should educate their children regarding the harmful effects of alcohol and drug abuse and provide proper knowledge and counseling regarding the consequences of addiction to drug and alcohol.
  (iii) Youngsters should be kept away from the company of friends who consume drugs.
  (iv) Children should be encouraged to devote their energy in other extra- curricular and recreational activities.
  (v) Regular and proper professional and medical consultation should be provided to a child if sudden symptoms of depression and frustration are observed.

9 Chapter
STRATEGIES FOR ENHANCEMENT IN FOOD PRODUCTION

CHAPTER AT A GLANCE

- The strategies for enhancement in food production aim at
  - increasing the amount of food obtained from animals.
  - increasing the yield of agricultural crops.

  For the above purposes, several methods have been developed which can be broadly grouped as – animal breeding and plant breeding.

ANIMAL HUSBANDRY

- **Animal husbandry** deals with the care, breeding & management of domesticated animals (called **livestocks**) that are useful to humans.
- These livestock are important in human welfare in the following ways:
  - They are responsible for production of milk through cattle breeding.
  - Increased production of eggs through poultry farming.
  - Improvement of quality of meat through fish farming.
  - These livestock help in the proper utilisation of animal wastes, e.g. production of biogas and manure from the dung.
  - Through bee keeping or apiculture, they produce more honey and bee wax.
- Animals used in animal husbandry are cattle, pig, sheep, poultry, fish and honeybees.
- Animal husbandry consists of several practices, including dairy farming, poultry farming, fisheries and apiculture (bee keeping).
- **In dairy farming**, those animals are housed from which we obtain milk and milk products. Milk yield is primarily dependent on the quality of breeds in the farm.
- **Poultry** is a rearing of domesticated fowls (chickens), ducks, geese, turkeys, guinea fowls and pigeons. These birds and their eggs are used as food.
- Poultry birds exclusively grown for meat are called *broilers*, *layers* are for egg production, *cockerel* for young male fowls and *rooster* are mature male fowls.
- Poultry were the last major group of food animals to be domesticated.
- **Fishery** is an industry devoted to the rearing, breeding, catching and marketing of fishes. Besides fishes, other aquatic animals like prawn, crab etc. are also included.

- **Pisciculture** is the rearing, breeding and catching of fishes.
- **Aquaculture** is rearing and management of useful aquatic plants and animals like fishes, oysters, mussels and prawns etc.
- Fishes are reared and caught for food which is rich in proteins, vitamins A and D. Marine animals are also richer in iodine. Shark liver oil and cod liver oil are very good source of vitamins A and D.
- **Apiculture** is rearing and breeding of honeybees for the production of honey.
- The **commonest species of honeybee** is *Apis indica*.
- Honeybees have **three social castes**, each with a specific role or set of roles. These are **queen, worker bee and drones**.
- Hives produce 5 distinct substances: **honey, beeswax, propolis, pollen, and royal jelly**.

Animal Breeding

- **Animal breeding** is the production of new breeds of domesticated animals with improved traits.
- Improvement in genetic material is brought about by selective mating.
- Reduction in fertility after 4 – 6 matings is called **inbreeding depression**. This is overcome by breeding the superior animal with the animal of an unrelated breed.
- **Out-breeding** is the mating between the animals which are not closely related.
- **Cross-breeding** is the mating between the superior animals of different breeds of the same species.
- Cross breeding permits the desirable qualities of two different breeds to be combined. *Hisardale* is a new breed of sheep developed in Punjab by crossing Bikaneri ewes and Marino rams.
- **Interspecific hybridisation** is the mating between the animals of two different species. Mule is produced by mating between male ass and female horse (mare).
- **Hybrid vigour** is the superiority of hybrid in traits over either of its parents. It is also known as heterosis.
- **Artificial insemination** is a reproductive technology in which semen of a selected male artificially deposited into the vagina of a selected female.
- **MOET (Multiple Ovulation Embryo Transfer)** technique is a programme which improves the chances of successful production of hybrids.

PLANT BREEDING

- **Plant breeding** refers to the modification and improvement of genetic material of plants resulting in the development of crops which are more beneficial to human beings.
- It involves the production of a new variety with the desired characteristics such as resistance to diseases, climatic adaptability, and better productivity.
- There are different methods to produce desired variety of plants. The most common method of plant breeding is hybridisation
- **Hybridisation** is defined as the process of mixing of genome of two organisms to produce organism with new trait. Such plants with modified genome are known as **transgenic plants**.

- India is **mainly an agricultural country**. Agriculture accounts for approximately 33 per cent of India's GDP and employs nearly 62 per cent of the population.
- **Steps involved in plant breeding** are as follows:
  - **Collection of genetic variability.**
  - **Evaluation of germplasm and selection of parents.**
  - **Cross-hybridisation or breeding between selected parents.**
  - **Selection of superior hybrids.**
  - **Testing, release, and commercialization of new cultivars.**
- **Disease resistance** is the ability of plants to withstand, oppose, lessen or overcome the attack of pathogen.
- In 1963, several varieties such as **Sonalika and Kalyan Sona**, which were high yielding and disease resistant, were introduced all over the wheat-growing belt of India.
- Semi-dwarf rice varieties were derived from **IR-8, and Taichung Native-1were introduced in 1966**. Later better-yielding semi-dwarf varieties **Jaya and Ratna were developed in India**.
- *Saccharum barberi* and *Saccharum officinarum* were crossed to get the desirable qualities of high yield, thick stems, high sugar and ability to grow in the sugar cane areas of north India.
- Hybrid maize, jowar and bajra have been developed in India, which are high yielding and resistant to water stress.
- **Conventional breeding** is often constrained by the availability of limited number of disease resistance genes that are present and identified in various crop varieties or wild relatives. Inducing mutations in plants through diverse means and then screening the plant materials for resistance sometimes leads to desirable genes being identified.
- **Mutational breeding** is one of the methods of plant breeding that modifies base sequence/nucleotide sequence of a gene to obtain new traits other than those observed in parents. These mutations or changes are brought about either by chemicals or radiations such as X-rays.

  For example: Mung bean variety is obtained through mutation. This variety is resistant to "yellow mosaic virus".
- The **term mutation breeding** was first **coined by Freisleben and Lein in 1944** to refer the deliberate induction and development of mutant lines for crop improvement.
- **Pusa Lerma and Sharbati Sonora** are the two **important varieties of wheat produced by gamma ray's** treatment of Lerma Roja 64 (Mexican dwarf wheat varieties) and Sonora 64.
- **Dr Swaminathan** is called the **father of green revolution**. He has produced Sharbati Sonora, a variety of wheat by mutation which is responsible for green revolution in India.

- Green revolution refers to increase in production of food grains (such as rice and wheat) due to the introduction of high-yielding varieties, use of pesticides, and better management techniques.
- **Green revolution** is achieved through introductions of high yielding variety, increased irrigation facilities, fertilisers applications, weed, pest and better agricultural managements.
- **Biofortification** is the improvement of nutritional quality of crops to improve public health.
- In plant breeding, biofortification aims at developing new crops with improved
  - protein content and quality.
  - lipid content and quality.
  - vitamin and mineral content.
- It can be done either through selective breeding or genetic modification. This is employed to improve the content of proteins, oil, vitamins, minerals, and micro-nutrients in crops.
- There are several improved varieties of crop plants such as wheat, rice, maize, carrots, spinach etc. which have more nutritious value and more nutrients than the existing varieties.
- **Bioremediation** is a waste management technique that involves the use of organisms to remove or neutralize pollutants from a contaminated site.
- **Single cell protein** refers to the dried microbial cells or total protein extracted from pure microbial cell culture (algae, bacteria, yeasts and filamentous fungi) which can be used as food supplement to humans or animal.
- **Pruteen was the first commercial single cell protein** and was mainly used as animal feed supplement.
- Some **common microbes used as SCP producers** are as follows:
  - Bacteria-*Methylophillus*, *Methylotrophus*, *Brevibacterium*
  - Cyanobacteria-*Spirulina*
  - Yeast-*Saccharomyces cerevisiae*, *Candida utilize*
  - Filamentous fungi-*Fusarium graminearum*
  - Algae-*Chlorella*
- **Advantages of SCP**
  - Microorganisms show rapid growth, so it can be grown in a large amount in a small period of time.
  - We can grow on a wide range of raw materials and can be easily harvested.
  - We have relatively higher protein content as compared to other healthy food items
- Somatic hybridization was **first introduced by Carlson in *Nicotiana glauca***.
- **Gottlieb Haberlandth started the technique of plant tissue culture** in 1902.
- The term pure line was introduced by W. L. Johannsen in 1903. It is applicable to self-pollinated crops.
- The wheat variety HUW 468 is a good example of pure line.
- **Plant tissue culture** is defined as the maintenance and growth of plant cells, tissues and organs on a suitable culture medium *in vitro*.

- The part of the plant cultured is called **explant**.
- Explant may be excised root tips, shoot bud, leaf petiole, inflorescence, anther, ovule, ovary or embryo.
- **Embryoids** are embryo-like structures derived from vegetative cells.
- Plants thus produced are genetically identical to the original plant (**somaclones**).
- **Transgenic plants** are plants developed from the cells in which a particular gene has been transferred.
- **Haploid production** is the production of plants with cells having one genome. Culture of fused protoplasts produces somatic hybrid cells and the process of producing somatic hybrids are called **somatic hybridisation**.
- In **embryo culture** embryos taken out from seeds and grown on culture medium.

EXERCISE

1. Explain in brief the role of animal husbandry in human welfare.

Sol. Animal husbandry is the agricultural practice for caring, feeding, breeding and management of livestock by applying scientific principles. Livestock includes animals like buffaloes, cows, pigs, horses, cattle, sheep, camels, goats, etc., that are useful to humans. It includes poultry farming and fisheries. *Animal husbandry is important for human welfare* as:

(i) The ever-increasing demand of food from animals and animal products both in terms of quality and quantity has been met by good animal husbandry practices.

(ii) In view of the high nutritive value of honey and its medicinal importance, there has been a remarkable growth in the practice of bee-keeping or apiculture.

(iii) Fishery is another flourishing industry meeting the ever-increasing demand for fish, fish products and other aquatic foods.

(iv) These livestock help in the proper utilisation of animal wastes, e.g., production of biogas and manure from the dung.

(v) They provide products which are used as food like meat, milk, eggs, honey, etc.

(vi) There are some other substances obtained from animals which are beneficial to human beings like wool, silk, leather, bees wax, etc.

2. If your family owned a dairy farm, what measures would you undertake to improve the quality and quantity of milk production?

Sol. To improve the quality and quantity of milk production, one should undertake the following measures:

(i) Proper feeding of the cattle with good quality and quantity of food.

(ii) Stringent clean and hygienic environment for housing the cattles.

(iii) Proper medication.

(iv) Supply of adequate water.
(v) Stringent cleanliness and hygienic conditions while milking, storage and transport of milk and its products.
(vi) Regular inspection.
(vii) Veterinary supervision at regular intervals.
(viii) Selection of good breeds having high yielding capacity combined with resistance to disease.
(ix) Quality of breed.

3. What is meant by the term 'breed'? What are the objectives of animal breeding?

Sol.
- *Breed* refers to a group of animals which are related by descent to each other and similar in characteristics like appearance, size, features, etc.
- The *objectives of animal breeding* are:
  (i) Increasing the yield of animal produce such as milk, meat, egg, wool, etc.,
  (ii) Improving the desirable qualities of the produce, *i.e.,* superior quality of milk, meat, eggs, wool, etc.,
  (iii) Improving growth rate, resistance to various diseases and reproduction rate.
  (iv) Increasing productive life.

4. Name the methods employed in animal breeding. According to you which of the methods is best? Why?

Sol. Animal breeding is the process of selectively mating two animals of the same or different breeds with desired traits to maintain or enhance these traits in future generations.

- Various *methods employed in animal breeding* are:
  (i) *Inbreeding* : It is the mating of more closely related individuals within the same breed for 4 to 6 generations.
  (ii) *Out-breeding* : It is the breeding of the unrelated animals, which may be between individuals of the same breed but having no common ancestors for 4 to 6 generations (out-crossing) or between different breeds (cross-breeding) or different species (inter-specific hybridisation).
  (iii) *Out-crossing* : This is the practice of mating of animals within the same breed, but having no common ancestors on either side of their pedigree up to 4 to 6 generations. The offspring of such a mating is known as an out-cross.
  (iv) *Cross-breeding* : In this method, superior males of one breed are mated with superior females of another breed.
  (v) *Interspecific hybridisation* : In this method, male and female animals of two different related species are mated.

(vi) *Artificial insemination* : It is a controlled breeding experiment in which semen is collected from the male that is chosen as a parent and injected into the reproductive tract of the selected female by the breeder. The semen may be used immediately or can be frozen and used at a later date. It can also be transported in a frozen form to where the female is housed. In this way, desirable matings are carried.

(vii) *Multiple Ovulation Embryo Transfer Technology* (MOET) : In this method, a cow is administered hormones, with FSH-like activity, to induce follicular maturation and superovulation so they produce 6 to 8 eggs. The animal is either mated with an elite bull or artificially inseminated. The fertilised eggs at 8-32 cells stages, are recovered non-surgically and transferred to surrogate mothers. The genetic mother is available for another round of super ovulation.

- *Cross breeding is the best method* as it results in the development of superior traits of both the breeds and the progeny produced are fertile and there is no inbreeding depression.

Note

Inbreeding depression is the reduced biological fitness in a given population as a result of inbreeding.

5. What is apiculture? How is it important in our lives?

Sol.
- *Apiculture*, also called bee-keeping, is the rearing and breeding of honeybees for the production of honey.
- *Apiculture is important* for us in the following ways:
  (i) It provides honey which is a food of high nutritive value and also finds use in the indigenous systems of medicine.
  (ii) It also produces beeswax, which finds many uses in industry, such as in the preparation of cosmetics and polishes of various kinds.
  (iii) Bees are the pollinators of many crop plants such as sunflower, *Brassica*, apple and pear. Keeping beehives in crop fields, during flowering period, increases pollination efficiency and improves both crop yield and honey yield.

6. Discuss the role of fishery in enhancement of food production.

Sol. Fishery is a practice of rearing, catching, processing or selling of fish, shellfish or other aquatic animals. A large part of human population is dependent on fish, fish products and other aquatic animals such as prawn, crab, lobster, edible oyster, etc., for food. In order to meet the increasing demands on fisheries, different techniques have been employed to increase the production of aquatic plants and animals, both fresh-water and marine through aquaculture and pisciculture. Also, fishes and sea food rich in protein and high nutrition value has also been produced.

7. Briefly describe various steps involved in plant breeding.

Sol. Plant breeding is the purposeful manipulation of plant species in order to create desired plant types that are better suited for cultivation, give better yields and are disease resistant.

- *Steps involved in plant breeding*. The breeding of a new genetic variety of a crop involves the following steps:
  (i) *Collection of variability* : Firstly, all the different wild varieties, species and relatives of the cultivated species are collected and preserved. This entire collection in the form of plants or seeds having all the diverse alleles for all genes in a given crop is called germplasm collection. Germplasm collection has all the possible genetic variation which is the source of raw material for selection.
  (ii) *Evaluation and selection of parents* : After collection of germplasm, it is evaluated and plants with desirable combination of characters are identified as parents. The selected parent plants are multiplied and pure lines are created wherever desirable and possible.
  (iii) *Cross hybridisation among the selected parents* : In this step, selected parents with desirable characters are cross hybridised through artificial hybridisation to produce hybrids.
  (iv) *Selection and testing of superior recombinants* : During this step, hybrid plants with desired character combination are selected through careful scientific evaluation of the progeny. The selected hybrid plants are self-pollinated for several generations to reach a state of uniformity (homozygosity), so that the characters will not segregate in the progeny.
  (v) *Testing, release and commercialisation of new cultivars* : The newly selected lines are grown in research fields under ideal fertiliser application, irrigation, and other crop management practices and then evaluated for their yield and other agronomic traits of quality, disease resistance, etc. This is followed by testing the materials in farmers' fields, for at least three growing seasons at several locations in the country, representing all the agroclimatic zones where the crop is usually grown. The material is evaluated in comparison to the best available local crop cultivar - a check or reference cultivar.

8. Explain what is meant by biofortification.

Sol.
- *Biofortification* is the breeding of crops for improved nutritional quality through both conventional plant breeding and recombinant DNA technology (genetic engineering).
- It is undertaken to increase both bioavailability and the concentration of nutrients in crops *i.e.*, for improved content and quality of protein, oil, vitamin, micronutrient and minerals. It is a cost-effective, feasible means of delivering micronutrients to populations who may have limited access to diverse diets, supplements, or commercially fortified foods. Thus, it is a practical means to improve public health.

- Some of the examples of biofortified crops are Atlas 66, a wheat variety having a high protein content, an iron-fortified rice variety, vitamin A enriched carrots, spinach and pumpkin, vitamin C enriched bitter gourd, bathua, mustard, tomato, iron and calcium enriched spinach and bathua and protein enriched broad bean, lablab, French and garden peas.

9. Which part of the plant is best suited for making virus-free plants and why?

Sol.
- Shoot and root apical meristems and axillary meristem can be used to obtain virus-free plants.
- The meristems are free of virus even if the plant is infected with a virus. Hence, one can remove the meristem and grow it *in vitro* to obtain virus-free plants.

10. What is the major advantage of producing plants by micropropagation?

Sol. Micropropagation is a method of producing a large number of plants through tissue culture.

Major advantages of this method are as follows:

(i) A large number of plants are propagated in very short durations.

(ii) Micropropagated plants are genetically identical to the original plant from which they were grown. Thus, desired traits can be maintained generation after generation.

(iii) It is possible to recovery of healthy plants from diseased plants by this method.

(iv) It gives propagules for plant multiplication throughout irrespective of the season.

(v) It requires small part of plant called explant and less space to generate the whole plants.

(vi) Genetically modified cells or cells after protoplast fusion can be multiplied through this method.

11. Find out the various components of the medium used for propagation of an explant *in vitro*?

Sol. The nutrient medium used for propagation of explants *in vitro* must have the following components:

(i) A carbon source such as sucrose

(ii) Inorganic salts

(iii) Vitamins

(iv) Amino acids

(v) Growth regulators like auxins, cytokinins

12. Name any five hybrid varieties of crop plants which have been developed in India.

Sol. Five hybrid varieties of crop plants developed in India are:

S. No.	Crop plant	Variety
1.	Wheat	Himgiri (resistant to leaf and stripe rust, hill bunt)
2.	Rice	Jaya and Ratna (High yielding dwarf variety)
3.	*Brassica*	Pusa swarnim (Karan rai) (resistant to white rust)
4.	Cowpea	Pusa Komal (resistant to bacterial blight)
5.	Chili	Pusa Sadabahar (resistant to chilly mosaic virus, tobacco mosaic virus and leaf curl)

Chapter 10 MICROBES IN HUMAN WELFARE

CHAPTER AT A GLANCE

- **Microbes** are various – bacteria, fungi, protozoa, bacteria, fungi and minute plants viruses, viroids furthermore prions (proteinaceous agents of infection).
- Microbes are present everywhere that is in soil, water, air, inside the body of plants and animals, inside thermal vents, deep in the soil, under the layers of snow several meters thick and in highly acidic environments.
- Microbes can be grown on culture nutritive media to form colonies which are used for mass production of certain desirable products and for scientific study of metabolism, genetics and structure of micro-organism.

MICROBES AND THEIR ROLES

- **LAB** is lactic acid bacteria which produce acids that coagulates and partially digest the milk proteins. Milk is changed into curd, yoghurt & cheese etc.
- **Louis Pasteur** discovered fermentation in 1857.
- The dough, which is used for making foods such as dosa and idli is **fermented by bacteria**. The puffed-up appearance of dough is due to the production of **CO_2 gas** which is released by the microbes.
- Similarly, the dough, which is used for making bread, is fermented using **baker's yeast** (*Saccharomyces cerevisiae*).
- A number of traditional drinks and foods are also made by fermentation by the microbes. **'Toddy'**, a traditional drink of some parts of southern India is made by fermenting sap from palms.
- **Ethanol**, also called ethyl alcohol, is the alcohol found in alcoholic beverages. It is produced by fermenting sugars with yeast (*Saccharomyces cerevisiae*).
- **Antibiotics** are chemical substances, which are produced by some microbes and can kill or retard growth of other disease causing microbes.
- Penicillin was the **first antibiotic to be discovered**. Alexander Fleming while working on *Staphylococci* plates observed that in one of unwashed culture plate, it could not grow because of chemical produced by mould *Penicilliun notatum* grown on it which produces chemical **penicillin**.
- Antibiotics have been extensively used for treatment of certain epidemic diseases like cough, diphtheria, leprosy, plague, etc.

- Examples of **acid producers** are ***Aspergillus niger*** (a fungus) of citric acid, ***Acetobacter aceti*** (a bacterium) of acetic acid, ***Clostridium butylicum*** (a bacterium) of butyric acid, ***Lactobacillus*** (a bacterium) of **lactic acid**, ***Saccharomyces*** *cerevisiae* of lactic acid etc.
- **Streptokinase**, produced by bacterium *Streptococcus*, is used as clot buster for removing blood clot in patients suffering from myocardial infractions.
- **Cyclosporin A** is a bioactive immunosuppressive agent and used in organ transplant patient. It is produced by *Trichoderma polysporum*.
- **Statin** is blood cholesterol lowering agent produced by yeast *Monascus* and it acts by competitively inhibiting enzyme responsible for cholesterol synthesis.
- *Thiobacillus thiooxidans* and *thiobacillus ferroxidans*, when grown in presence of copper ore produce acid and affect oxidation process known as **leaching** and improves recovery of metal from ore and is non-polluting to the atmosphere.
- **Wastewater treatment** process are carried out by municipal treatment plant as a community process. These are **primary treatment & secondary treatment**.
- **Primary (1°) Treatment :** This is a physical process that involves physical removal of particles from the sewage through filtration and sedimentation. So, it remove coarse solids and settleable solids in sedimentation units (tanks, basin, or mechanical devices) by which particulate material is concentrated as **sludge**. The sludge and liquid effluent are processed separately. The effluent from the primary settling tank is taken to secondary treatment.
- **Secondary (2°) treatment :** This treatment involves the oxidation of organic material in effluent by microbial method. These are –
  - Activated sludge process.
  - **Filteration** by intermittent sand filters and trickling filter.
- **In activated sludge process,** aeration of sewage in large aeration and agitation tank, lead to the formation of **flocs** (masses of bacteria associated with fungal filaments to form mesh like structure) and floccules. When they are vigorously aerated, flocculation occurs and this contain large number of actively metabolising bacteria, yeast, mould and protozoa. This growth is effective in oxidation of organic compound. This significantly reduces BOD (Biochemical oxygen demand).
- **BOD** refers to the amount of the oxygen that would be consumed if all the organic matter in one liter of water were oxidised by bacteria.
- The sewage water is treated till the BOD is reduced. **BOD is a measure of the organic matter present in the water**. The greater the BOD of waste water, more is its polluting potential.

- **Anaerobic sludge digester :** Solid which accumulates during sedimentation are pumped into sludge digester. This sludge is digested with the help of anaerobic and facultative bacteria. These micro-organisms bring about a decrease in organic solid by degrading them to soluble substances and gaseous products which has 60-70% methane and 20-30% CO_2. This gas mixture is used as **biogas** for heating purpose and for operating power.
- **Composting** is decomposition of dewatered sludge by thermophilic bacteria under forced aeration. Effective period of time is 21 days after which it transforms into humus type material and is suitable for use as a soil conditioner.

MICROBES IN BIOGAS PRODUCTION

- **Biogas** is a gaseous fuel, produced by methanogens, which are anaerobic bacteria growing on cellulosic material and produce large amount of methane alongwith CO_2 and H_2, e.g., *Methanococcus, Methanobacterium.*
- Biogas plant works based on the process called anaerobic digestion or fermentation of organic matter including manure, sewage sludge, municipal solid waste, biodegradable waste or any other biodegradable feedstock under anaerobic conditions.

MICROBES AS BIOCONTROL AGENT AND BIOFERTILISERS

- Use of predators, animal composite, micro-organisms such as bacteria/virus to control insect pest, pathogen and weed is called **biological control** and biological agents are called **biocontrol agents**.
- **Bt cotton** is genetically modified cotton having *Bacillus thuringiensis* genes. Bacterium *Bacillus thuringiensis* (Bt) is used as microbial control agent in order to control butterfly caterpillars. It is sprayed on plants like *Brassica* and fruit trees which are attacked by insect larvae. *Bt* release toxin and insect larvae are killed. It is killing only caterpillars, leaving all other insects unharmed.
- **Biofertilisers** are organisms that enrich nutrient quality of soil. The main source is bacteria, fungi and cyanobacterium.

  Examples :
  - *Rhizobium* species in root nodules of leguminous plant.
  - *Azospirillium* and *Azotobacter* are free living species in soil.
  - **Fungi** : *Glomus* in symbiotic association with plant where fungal symbiont absorb phosphorus from soil and passes to plants. Plants inturn show better resistance to root borne pathogens, tolerance to salinity and draught, overall growth of plant.
  - **Cyanobacteria** such as *Anabaena*, *Nostoc* and *Oscillatoria* (autotrophic microbes) in paddy field.
- In paddy fields, cyanobacteria serve as an important biofertiliser. Blue green algae also add organic matter to the soil and increase its fertility.
- **Organic farming** is use of biofertilisers, biocontrol agents and biologically produced compost.

EXERCISE

1. Bacteria cannot be seen with the naked eyes, but these can be seen with the help of a microscope. If you have to carry a sample from your home to your biology laboratory to demonstrate the presence of microbes under a microscope, which sample would you carry and why?

Sol. Bacteria are microscopic single-celled organisms that thrive in diverse environments. They cannot be seen with the naked eyes, but these can be seen with the help of a microscope.

Sample which is easy to carry from home to biology laboratory for the study of microbes present in them is curd because curd contains lactobacilli bacteria.

Curd is formed from milk. A small drop of curd contains millions of lactic acid bacteria (LAB) or *Lactobacillus*, which can be easily observed under a microscope. The curd forms because of the chemical reaction between the lactic acid bacteria and casein (present in milk along with lactose, a disachharide sugar). During fermentation, the bacteria use enzymes to produce energy (ATP) from lactose. The by-product of ATP production is lactic acid that coagulates and digests milk proteins.

> **Note**
>
> *The species of bacteria used in yogurt are Streptococcus thermophilus and Lactobacillus bulgaricus. These species eat the sugars in milk. As the bacteria eat milk sugars, the bacteria produce lactic acid.*

2. Give examples to prove that microbes release gases during metabolism.

Sol. Microbial metabolism is the means by which a microbe obtains the energy and nutrients (e.g. carbon) it needs to live and reproduce.

Microbes that release gases during metabolism in the given process are as follows:

(i) *Fermentation* : Bacteria and fungi carry out the process of fermentation and during this process, they release carbon dioxide. Fermentation is the process of converting a complex organic substance into a simpler substance with the action of bacteria or yeast. Fermentation of sugar produces alcohol with the release of carbon dioxide and very little energy.

$$\text{Glucose} \xrightarrow[\text{oxygen}]{\text{without}} \text{Alcohol} + \text{Energy} + CO_2$$

(ii) *Indian food* : The dough used for making idli and dosa gives a puffed appearance. This is because of the action of bacteria which releases carbon dioxide (CO_2) gas. This carbon dioxide gets trapped in the dough, thereby giving it a puffed appearance.

(iii) *Sewage treatment* : During secondary treatment of sewage in sewage treatment plants, a number of gases like methane are produced during microbial digestion of organic compounds.

3. In which food would you find lactic acid bacteria? Mention some of their useful applications.

Sol. Lactic acid bacteria (LAB) are among the most important groups of microorganisms used in food fermentations. They contribute to the taste and texture of fermented products and inhibit food spoilage bacteria by producing growth-inhibiting substances and large amounts of lactic acid.

- *As agents of fermentation LAB are involved* in making curd, yogurt, cheese, cultured butter, sour cream, sausage, cucumber pickles, olives and sauerkraut, but some species may spoil beer, wine and processed meats.
- *Application of lactic acid bacteria*
  (i) It plays an important role in curdling of milk. Under suitable condition, these bacteria multiply and produce acids (lactic acid) which coagulate and partially digest the milk proteins and change the milk into curd.
  (ii) It also increases the content of vitamin B_{12} in curd.
  (iii) They are also found in the human stomach where these bacteria prevent the growth of certain disease-causing microbes.

Note

- *Because LAB obtains energy only from the metabolism of sugars, they are restricted to environments in which sugars are present.*
- *Curd is a good source of vitamin B_{12}. Milk is also source of vitamin B_{12} but while formation of curd its concentration increases due the fact that lactobacilli synthesise vitamin B_{12}.*

4. Name some traditional Indian foods made of wheat, rice and Bengal gram (or their products) which involve use of microbes.

Sol. Traditional Indian foods made by microbes are as follows:

- Wheat : Bread, Bhatura, Jalebi, Cake etc.
- Rice : Idli, Dosa, Nan etc.
- Bengal gram : Dhokla, Khandavi etc.

5. In which way have microbes played a major role in controlling diseases caused by harmful bacteria?

Sol. Microbes are microscopic organism which include bacteria, protozoa, some fungi and algae. Some microbes play an important role in our daily lives by keeping us healthy while some are disease-causing microbes (called pathogens) and can make humans, animals and plants sick by causing infection and disease.

- Still *microbes play an important role in controlling diseases* (caused by harmful bacteria) by producing antibiotics. Antibiotics is a drug produced by one microorganisms that selectivily inhibits the growth of another.
  Antibiotics either kill or retard the growth of disease-causing microbes. They destroy bacteria by weakening their cell walls as a result of which certain immune cells such as the white blood cells enter the bacterial cell and cause cell lysis. These medicines are commonly obtained from bacteria and fungi.
  Example of antibiotics are streptomycin, tetracycline, and penicillin.
  So, antibiotics are being used in controlling a number of bacterial diseases like cholera, pneumonia, typhoid, syphilis, whooping cough, diphtheria etc.

Note

Antibiotics cannot control infections caused by viruses, such as colds, flu, most coughs and bronchitis, sore throats.

6. **Name any two species of fungus, which are used in the production of the antibiotics.**

Sol. Antibiotics are medicines that are produced by certain micro-organisms (bacteria and fungi) to kill other disease-causing micro-organisms. The species of fungus used in the production of antibiotics are given in the table below.

S. No.	Fungus species	Antibiotics
1.	*Penicillium notatum*	Penicillin
2.	*Penicillium griseofulvin*	Griseofulvin
3.	*Cephalosporium acremonium*	Cephalosporin

7. **What is sewage? In which way can sewage be harmful to us?**

Sol.
- *Sewage* is the municipal waste water containing human excreta which flows through the sewers. It includes both liquid and solid wastes, rich in organic matter and microbes.
- *Sewage can be harmful to us* in the following ways:
  (i) As it contains large amount of biodegradable organic matter which when decomposed by naturally occurring microbes in the presence of oxygen, then there is sharp decline in dissolved oxygen (DO). This causes suffocation of large number of aquatic animals like prawns, fishes, etc. Such waters become unfit for human consumption.
  (ii) It is a major cause of polluting drinking water. Hence, it is essential that sewage water is properly collected, treated, and disposed.
  (iii) It decreases flora and fauna of the water.
  (iv) Sewage contains pathogenic micro-organisms which are responsible for causing diseases like cholera, typhoid, dysentery, hepatitis, etc.

8. What is the key difference between primary and secondary sewage treatment?

Sol. Sewage treatment is the process of removing contaminants from municipal wastewater containing mainly household sewage plus some industrial wastewater. There are three stages of sewage treatment: primary, secondary and tertiary.

Key difference between primary and secondary sewage treatment are as follows:

S. No.	Primary sewage treatment	Secondary sewage treatment
1.	It is a physical process of screening, comminuting, grit removal, and sedimentation.	It is a biological process involving the action of microbes. Microbes consume the organic impurities as food, converting them into carbon dioxide, water, and energy for their own growth and reproduction.
2.	It is involved in the removal of coarse particles that will either float or readily settle out by gravity.	It removes the soluble organic matter that escapes primary treatment. It also removes more of the suspended solids. Sedimentation of bacterial flocs is done to aerobic sludge digesters for digestion.
3.	It is inexpensive and relatively less complicated.	It is a very expensive and complicated process.

9. Do you think microbes can also be used as source of energy? If yes, how?

Sol.
- Yes, microbes can be used as a source of energy in the form of biogas (or gobar gas).
  Microbes can be used extensively to produce biogas/gobar gas from animal dung (gobar) that is used as fuel in rural areas. The major component of biogas is methane (about 50–68%) which is highly inflammable. The other gases are hydrogen (25–35%), nitrogen (1–5%), oxygen (2–7%) and (traces) (0–0.1%).
- *Process of biogas generation* : Bacteria such as methanobacterium are used for the generation of gobar gas or biogas. Biogas is produced from degradable organic matter by the activity of various anaerobic microorganisms present in cow dung. The dung is mixed with water to form the slurry and thrown into the tank. The digester of the tank is filled with numerous anaerobic methane-producing bacteria, which produce biogas from the slurry. Biogas can be removed through the pipe which is then used as a source of energy, while the consumed slurry is removed from the outlet and is used as a fertiliser.
  Biogas produced is used as fuel for heating and cooking, lighting, power for irrigation and other purposes as an alternative of fire wood, kerosene, dung cakes or even electricity and LPG. It is considered as ecofriendly and pollution free source of energy.

10. Microbes can be used to decrease the use of chemical fertilisers and pesticides. Explain how this can be accomplished.

Sol. • Microbes *play an important role in organic farming*. Organic farming is a farming method that involves growing and nurturing crops without the use of chemical fertilisers and pesticides. It can be done by using biofertilisers.

Bio-fertilisers include those organisms that enrich the nutrient quality of the soil and help in improving plant growth through the supply of plant nutrients. The main sources of biofertilisers are bacteria, fungi and cyanobacteria.

Many species of bacteria and cyanobacteria have the ability to fix free atmospheric nitrogen.

Microbes used as biofertilisers are–

(i) *Azospirillum, Rhizobium* and *Azotobacter*: They can fix atmospheric nitrogen in the soil.

(ii) Blue green algae like *Anabaena, Nostoc* and *Oscillatoria* : They add organic matter to the soil and responsible to increase its fertility.

They can provide plant nutrients at cheaper cost when compared with the chemical fertilisers.

• *Biofertilisers can also act as bio-pesticides* to control insect pests in plants, e.g.

(i) *Bacillus thuringiensis*, which produces a toxin that kills the insect pests.

(ii) *Trichoderma*, free living fungi, live in the roots of higher plants and protect them from various pathogens.

(iii) Baculovirus is another bio-pesticide that is used as a biological control agent against insects and other arthropods.

11. Three water samples namely river water, untreated sewage water and secondary effluent discharged from a sewage treatment plant were subjected to BOD test. The samples were labelled A, B and C; but the laboratory attendant did not note which was which. The BOD values of the three samples A, B and C were recorded as 20mg/L, 8mg/L and 400mg/L, respectively. Which sample of the water is most polluted? Can you assign the correct label to each assuming the river water is relatively clean?

Hints

The greater the BOD of waste water more is its polluting potential.

Sol. Biochemical Oxygen Demand (BOD), as an important water quality parameter, is the amount of dissolved oxygen needed (*i.e.* demanded) by aerobic biological organisms to break down organic material present in a given water sample at certain temperature over a specific time period.

BOD values indicate the amounts of organic wastes present in the matter.

On the basis of the given information regarding the sample (A, B and C) and their BOD value as given in the table below, it can be concluded that water of sample C is most polluted and water of sample B is relatively clean.

Label	BOD value	Sample	Reason
A	20 mg/L	Secondary effluent discharge from a sewage treatment plant	Because it comes after the primary treatment and is with less organic matter than untreated sewage water so have fewer BODS (*i.e.,* 20 mg/L).
B	8 mg/L	River water	It has minimum BOD (*i.e.,* 8 mg/L) and it has been assumed that river water is relatively clean so B sample is of river water.
C	400 mg/L	Untreated sewage water	Because such sewage water has highest quantities of organic matter and so has highest BOD value (*i.e.,* 400 mg/L).

12. Find out the name of the microbes from which Cyclosporin A (an immunosuppressive drug) and Statins (blood cholesterol lowering agents) are obtained.

Sol. • *Cyclosporin A*

(i) It is produced by fungus *Trichoderma polysporum.*

(ii) It was the first immunosuppressant that acted selectively to suppress T-cell immunity.

• *Statins*

(i) It is a blood cholesterol lowering agents which are produced by yeast *Monascus purpureus.*

(ii) It helps lower the level of low-density lipoprotein (LDL) cholesterol in the blood. It may also help to reabsorb cholesterol that has built up in plaques on the artery walls and thereby preventing further blockage in the blood vessels and heart attacks.

13. Find out the role of microbes in the following and discuss it with your teacher.

(a) Single cell protein (SCP)

(b) Soil

Sol. (a) *Single cell protein (SCP)*

- Single cell protein refers to protein obtained from cells of certain microbes like yeast, fungi, algae and bacteria which are grown on various carbon sources for synthesis.
- It contains about 45–55% proteins and considered to be an ideal supplement to conventional human food supply and animal feeds.

- It can be used to solve the problem of protein deficiency in the children of developing countries.
- Most commonly employed bacterial strains to produce SCP are *Methylophillus*, *Paecilomyces*, *Chlorella*, *Spirullina*, etc.

(b) *Soil*

- Soil contains a number of useful as well as harmful microbes.
- Microbes play an important role in maintaining soil fertility and help in formation of nutrient-rich humus by decomposition.
- Many species of bacteria and cyanobacteria have the ability to fix atmospheric nitrogen into usable form. The economically useful bacteria included in the soil are:
  (i) Ammonifying bacteria: These bacteria decompose the proteins of dead organisms and nitrogenous wastes of animals to ammonia, e.g., *Bacillus ramous* and *B. vulgari*.
  (ii) Nitrifying bacteria: They oxidise ammonia to nitrites, e.g. *Nitrosomonas*, *Nitrobacter*, etc.
  (iii) Nitrates fixing bacteria: They fix the atmospheric nitrogen as ammonia by the reduction process, e.g., *Rhizobium*, *Azotobacter*, *Clostridium*, etc.

14. Arrange the following in the decreasing order (most important first) of their importance, for the welfare of human society. Give reasons for your answer.
Biogas, Citric acid, Penicillin and Curd

Sol. The order of arrangement of products according to their decreasing importance is:

Penicillin > Biogas > Curd > Citric acid.

It is so because of the following roles :

- *Penicillin* : It is commonly called as wonder drug. It is a wide-spectrum antibiotic and used to control a number of human diseases like syphilis, gonorrhoea, diphtheria, lung infections, etc. Hence, it is good for health of society.
- *Biogas* : It is produced from dung of cattle by the methanogens and considered as an alternative source of energy especially in the rural areas. It is an eco-friendly source of energy and its production also provides slurry which can be used as a manure to increase the soil fertility and crop yield. It is a renewable source and easily maintained and dissipated for community purpose.
- *Curd* : It is a milk product, commonly used in almost all the houses. It has only nutritious value. It is obtained by the action of *Lactobacillus* bacteria on milk.
- *Citric acid* : It is least important for society but can be used as a food preservative and as an excipient in pharmaceutical preparations due to its antioxidant properties.

15. How do biofertilisers enrich the fertility of the soil?

Sol. Bio-fertilisers are cost effective and eco-friendly. They are living organisms which help in increasing the fertility of soil as follows:

(i) It includes the selection of useful micro-organisms that help in improving the plant growth through the supply of plant nutrients.

(ii) These are introduced to seeds, roots, or soil to mobilise the availability of nutrients by their biological activity. Thus, they are extremely beneficial in enriching the soil with organic nutrients.

(iii) Many species of bacteria and cyanobacteria have the ability to fix free atmospheric nitrogen. For examples,

- *Rhizobium* : It is a symbiotic bacterium found in the root nodules of leguminous plants.
- *Azospirillium* and *Azotobocter* are free living nitrogen-fixing bacteria, whereas *Anabaena*, *Nostoc*, and *Oscillatoria* are examples of nitrogen-fixing cyanobacteria.

Chapter 11 BIOTECHNOLOGY : PRINCIPLES AND PROCESSES

CHAPTER AT A GLANCE

- **Biotechnology** is the application of techniques of using live organism to get desired product of human welfare. It includes recombinant DNA, gene cloning, gene therapy.
- Biotechnology deals with large scale production and marketing of products and processes using living organisms, cells or enzymes.
- **Examples of biotechnology** are GMO (Genetically modified organisms), IVF (*in vitro* fertilisation), Test tube babies, DNA vaccines and gene therapy.
- **Two main techniques** in biotechnology are –
  (i) Genetic engineering.
  (ii) Application of genetic engineering in production of bulk of products like antibiotics, vaccines and enzymes.
- **Genetic engineering** is manipulation of genes by man.
- Genetic engineering includes several techniques that facilitate the alteration of genetic material *i.e.* RNA or DNA, in order to introduce them in host organisms.
- **Paul berg** is the **father of genetic engineering**.
- **Enzymes used in genetic engineering** are restriction endonucleases, DNA ligase, exonuclease, endonuclease, DNA polymerase, and reverse transcriptase.
- **Three techniques** of genetic engineering are:
  (i) rDNA (recombinant DNA technology)
  (ii) Gene cloning/gene amplification
  (iii) Gene therapy
- **rDNA technology** is hybridisation of genes to achieve desired genotype and phenotype.
- **Tools of rDNA** technology are –
  (i) **Vector** – plasmid, bacteriophage, cosmid, BAC, YAC.
  (ii) **Host** – with Ori C [origin of replication].
  (iii) **Restriction enzymes** – Endonuclease with well defined recognition site.
- **Steps of rDNA technology** are :
  – Isolation of desired gene by cutting with molecular scissors called "restriction endonuclease".
  – Introduction of gene into vector (cloning vehicle).
  – Absorption of vector by host organism in culture media.
  – Production of transformed cells.
  – Screening of transformed cells for desired result.

- **Vectors** are cloning vehicles required to transfer DNA of interest from one organism to another. Vectors are grouped into bacterial plasmid, bacteriophage, cosmids & phasmids.
  - **Plasmid** is an autonomously replicating extra chromosomal genetic content present in the bacteria. It is different from the chromosomal DNA. It is used as a vehicle for transfer of gene of interest into the host cell.
  - **Bacteriophage** is virus which infect bacteria. They have special sticky "cos" site to accept foreign DNA. As bacteriophage multiply faster, so transformation efficiency is higher in bacteriophage.
  - **Cosmid** can be defined as the hybrid vectors derived from plasmids which contain *cos* site of phage 1.
  - A phage genome containing *att* site and one more plasmid molecule is called **phasmid**.
- **BAC** (Bacterial Artificial Chromosome) is episome + foreign DNA.
- **Palindromic sequences** are the ones which read same in one orientation on both the strands.

  For e.g., 5'—GAATTC—3'

  3'—CTTAAG—5'

  is palindrome as it reads same on both strands in 5' $\rightarrow$ 3' direction. Same is true for 3' $\rightarrow$ 5' direction.
- **Restriction endonuclease** cut DNA at specific sites end exonuclease digest the base pairs on 5' or 3' end of a single stranded DNA or at single stranded nicks or gaps in double stranded DNA.
- **Nomenclature of restriction endonuclease are–**

  1st letter – Generic name

  2nd letter – Species name

  3rd letter – Strain name

  4th letter – Order in which enzyme is isolated from that strain of bacteria [Roman Numeral] e.g., *EcoRY*13 $\rightarrow$ stands for ***Escherichia* coli** strain **RY numbered 13.**
- **Desirable properties of cloning vector** are –
  (i) High copy number
  (ii) Presence of origin of replication (Ori)
  (iii) Presence of selectable marker
  (iv) Presence of unique recognition site in cloning site
  (v) Ability to sustain in bacterial cell/low incompatibility quotient.
- **Ori C** is sequence where replication starts and any piece of DNA linked here will be replicated. Ori C also controls copy number of vector.
- **Selectable marker** allow to select those host cells that contain the vector from amongst those which do not.
- **For cloning :** First an artificial plasmid is synthesised by combining marker gene to it, e.g., **pUC 11** (plasmid developed at University of California) and **pBR 322.**

- *Agrobacterium tumefaciens* is cloning vector for plants which is **T-DNA** (transforming DNA), to transform normal plant cell into tumour and direct them to form mass of cells called **galls** which start secreting chemicals required by bacteria.

  In vitro synthesis of DNA of interest can be done by **PCR (polymerase chain reaction)**. In this reaction, multiple copies of the gene (or DNA) of interest is synthesised *in vitro* using two sets of primers (small chemically synthesised oligonucleotides that are complementary to the regions of DNA) and the enzyme DNA polymerase. The enzyme extends the primers using the nucleotides provided in the reaction and the genomic DNA as template.
- The product from rDNA can be obtained at large scale in **bioreactors** – where from an inlet, large volume of culture medium is fed and from an outlet, used media is thrown out.

  Bioreactor provide optimum conditions for achieving desired product by providing optimum growth conditions [temperature, pH, salt, sugar, vitamin].
- **Downstream processing** is separation and purification of products achived from bioreactors. The product is converted into formulation for usage, tested sfor human use, undergoes quality control and then marketed.

EXERCISE

1. Can you list 10 recombinant proteins which are used in medical practice? Find out where they are used as therapeutics (use the internet).

Sol. Recombinant proteins are the proteins that are produced through recombinant DNA technology. These proteins are produced from the expression of protein encoding gene in another organism after its transfer using vectors. *10 recombinant proteins used in medical practices and their therapeutic uses* are as follows:

S. No.	Recombinant proteins	Therapeutic uses
1.	Insulin	Treatment for type I diabetes mellitus
2.	Blood clotting factor VIII	Treatment of haemophilia A
3.	Blood clotting factor IX	Treatment of haemophilia B
4.	Alpha interferon	Used for chronic hepatitis C
5.	Interferon beta	For treatment of multiple sclerosis
6.	DNase I	Treatment of cystic fibrosis
7.	Anti-thrombin III	Prevention of blood clot
8.	Tissue plasminogen activator	Treatment of blood clot in acute myocardial infection
9.	Recombinant Human growth hormone	Treatment of growth disorders in children
10.	Hirudin	As anticoagulant

2. Make a chart (with diagrammatic representation) showing a restriction enzyme, the substrate DNA on which it acts, the site at which it cuts DNA and the product it produces.

Sol. Restriction enzymes are endonucleases which recognise a specific palindromic nucleotide sequences in the DNA (called recognition sites) and make cuts in each of the two strands of the double helix at specific points within their recognition sites. For example, *Bam*H1 is a restriction enzyme whose recognition site is 6 base pairs in length.

The following *chart showing the substrate DNA, the cleavage site and the restriction products of Bam*H1 is given below.

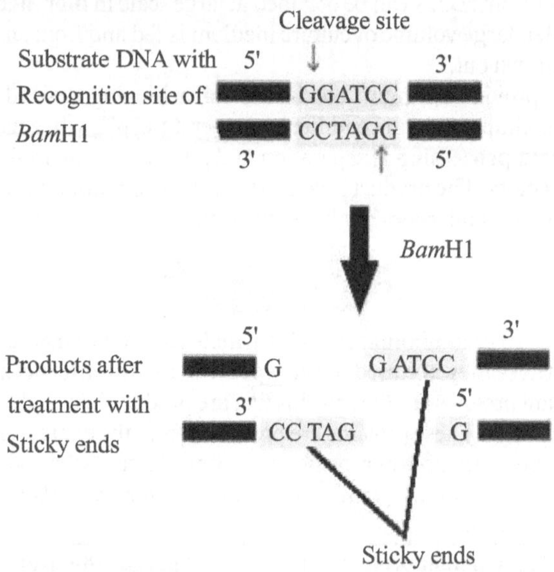

3. From what you have learnt, can you tell whether enzymes are bigger or DNA is bigger in molecular size? How did you know?

Sol.
- Though both DNA and enzymes are macromolecules, *DNA is bigger in molecular size* as compare to enzyme.
- This is because DNA is a polymer of deoxynucleotides and contains the information for the synthesis of proteins. In comparison, enzymes are proteins which are polymers of amino acids of variable number synthesised from a small segment of DNA called gene.

4. What would be the molar concentration of human DNA in a human cell? Consult your teacher.

Sol. The molar concentration of DNA is the molar concentration of the total nucleotides present in one human cell.

Genomic DNA per human cell = 6 picogram = 6×10^{-12} g

Average molar mass of a nucleotide = 327g/mol

Number of nucleotides in human genome = 6.6×10^{9}

Molar mass of haploid DNA $= 6.6 \times 10^9 \times 327$ g/mol $= 2158.2 \times 10^9$ g/mol

Number of moles of DNA in human cell $= 6 \times 10^{-12}$ g/2158.2 $\times 10^9$ g/mol

$= 27.8 \times 10^{-25}$ mol

Since genomic DNA is contained in nucleus,

Radius of nucleus $= 3\ \mu m = 3 \times 10^{-6}$ m

Volume of nucleus $= 4/3\ \pi\ (3 \times 10^{-6}\ m)^3$

$= 4/3\ \pi\ (3 \times 10^{-6}\ m)^3$

$= 113.14 \times 10^{-15}$ litres ($1 m^3 = 1000$ L)

$$\text{Molar concentration} = \frac{\textit{Number of moles of DNA}}{\textit{Volume of nucleus in litres}}$$

$$= \frac{27.8 \times 10^{-25}\ \text{mol}}{13.14 \times 10^{-15}\ \text{litres}}$$

$$= 2.46 \times 10^{-11} M$$

5. **Do eukaryotic cells have restriction endonucleases? Justify your answer.**

Sol.
- No, eukaryotic cells do not have restriction endonucleases.
- All the restriction endonucleases have been isolated from various strains of bacteria (prokaryotes). They possess these enzymes as a defence mechanism to destroy the foreign DNA or to restrict the growth of invading viruses called bacteriophages. Such mechanism to restrict the growth of invading viruses is absent in eukaryotes.

Note

DNA of eukaryotes is highly methylated by a modification enzyme, called methylase. Methylation protects the DNA from the activity of restriction enzymes.

6. **Besides better aeration and mixing properties, what other advantages do stirred tank bioreactors have over shake flasks?**

Sol.
- Shake flasks are used for growing and mixing the desired materials on a small scale in the laboratory. A large scale production of desired biotechnological products (100–1000 litres) is done by using 'bioreactors'. The most commonly used bioreactors are of stirring type. A stirred-tank reactor is usually cylindrical or with a curved base to facilitate the mixing of the reactor contents. The stirrer facilitates even mixing and oxygen availability throughout the bioreactor.
- Besides better aeration and mixing properties, *stirred tank bioreactors have following advantages*:
  - (i) It has sampling parts from where small volumes of cultures can be periodically withdrawn from the reactor for sampling.
  - (ii) It has a foam control system, pH control system and temperature control system.

7. Collect 5 examples of palindromic DNA sequences by consulting your teacher. Better try to create a palindromic sequence by following base-pair rules.

Sol. A palindromic DNA sequence is a sequence of base pairs that reads the same on the two strands when the orientation of reading of sequences in DNA is kept the same, *i.e.*, from 5'→3' or 3'→5'.

Five examples of palindromic DNA sequences are as follows:

(i) 5'——GTAC——3'
3'——CATG——5'

(ii) 5'——ATCGAT——3'
3'——TAGCTA——5'

(iii) 5'——ATGCAT——3'
3'——TACGTA——5'

(iv) 5'——CCGG——3'
3'——GGCC——5'

(v) 5'——ATTAAT——3'
3'——TAATTA——5'

8. Can you recall meiosis and indicate at what stage a recombinant DNA is made?

Hints

Third stage of Meiosis I, that is characterised by paired chromosomes thickened and visibly divided into chromatids and by the occurrence of crossing over.

Sol. Recombinant DNA is the DNA with new combination formed by the joining of two or more gene sequences. It is made during pachytene stage of prophase I of meiosis I. This is the stage when crossing over involving exchange of DNA segments between non-sister chromatids of homologous chromosomes takes place.

9. Can you think and answer how a reporter enzyme can be used to monitor transformation of host cells by foreign DNA in addition to a selectable marker?

Sol. Transformation is a procedure through which a piece of DNA is introduced in a host bacterium. Selectable markers are the genes present in vector that help in identification and elimination of non-transformants by selectively permitting the growth of the transformants. Genes encoding resistance to antibiotics such as ampicillin, chloramphenicol, tetracycline or kanamycin, etc., are examples of selectable markers.

Selection of recombinants due to inactivation of antibiotics is a cumbersome procedure because it requires simultaneous plating on two plates having different antibiotics. So gene encoding reporter enzyme linked to the gene of interest is used to monitor transformation of host cells. Such vectors have a reporter enzyme in addition to antibiotic resistance gene and recognition sites for restriction enzymes are present in gene encoding reporter enzyme. Reporter enzymes convert invisible substrates to luminescent or coloured products. Examples of reporter enzymes are β-galactosidase or alkaline phosphatase. If the bacteria transformed with vector without an insert, are grown on the medium containing substrate of β-galactosidase, blue coloured colonies are produced. If bacteria transformed with an insert within the coding sequence of β-galactosidase are grown on the medium containing substrate, the colonies do not produce any colour and form white colonies due to insertional inactivation of β-galactosidase. These white colonies are identified as recombinant colonies. Thus, on the basis of colour of colony, transformed host cells are selected.

Note

Use diagrammatic representation to understand the insertional inactivation of enzyme which is responsible for a coloured product. The visual will help in recall.

10. Describe briefly the followings:

(a) Origin of replication **(b) Bioreactors**

(c) Downstream processing

Sol. (a) Origin of replication (Ori)

Ori is a specific DNA sequence from where replication initiates and any piece of DNA when linked to this sequence can be made to replicate within the host cells. This sequence is also responsible for controlling the copy number of the linked DNA. So, if one wants to recover many copies of the target DNA it should be cloned in a vector whose origin support high copy number.

(b) Bioreactors

Bioreactors are vessels in which raw materials are biologically converted into specific products by microbes, plant and animal cell and/or their enzymes. The bioreactor provides optimum growth conditions for achieving the desired products. The most commonly used bioreactor is of stirring type. A stirred tank bioreactor is usually a cylindrical vessel or vessel with a curved base to facilitate mixing of the contents. In the sparged stirred tank bioreactor, sterile air bubbles are sparged. The stirrer facilitates the mixing and oxygen availability throughout the bioreactor. A bioreactor has an agitator system, an oxygen delivery system, a foam control system, a temperature control system, pH control system and sampling ports.

(c) Downstream processing

The product once obtained is subjected to a series of processes collectively called downstream processing before it is made into a finished product ready for marketing. The two main processes are separation and purification. The product is then formulated with suitable preservatives. Such formulations have to undergo clinical trials, in case of drugs. The downstream process and quality control test are different from product to product.

11. Explain briefly

(a) PCR **(b) Restriction enzymes and DNA**

(c) Chitinase

Sol. (a) PCR

- PCR or Polymerase chain reaction is a technique (developed by Kary Mullis in 1985) to synthesise multiple copies of gene or DNA of interest using a set of primers and DNA polymerase *in vitro*.
- Thermostable DNA polymerase, *Taq* DNA polymerase isolated from a bacterium, *Thermus aquaticus* is used in PCR. These enzyme remains active during the high temperature induced for denaturation of double-stranded DNA.

- The process of amplification of gene of interest using PCR technique involves following three steps:
  (i) *Denaturation* : In this step, reaction mixture heated to separate double-stranded template DNA into two single strands.
  (ii) *Annealing* : In this step, the reaction mixture is cooled so the primers can bind to their complementary sequences on the single-stranded template DNA strands.
  (iii) *Extension* : In this step, temperature of the reaction mixture is raised to 72°C so *Taq* polymerase extends the primers using the nucleotides provided in the reaction and the genomic DNA as template, synthesising new strands of DNA.

  These steps are repeated in a cyclic manner and the gene of interest is amplified to approximately billion times, *i.e.*, 1 billion copies are made.

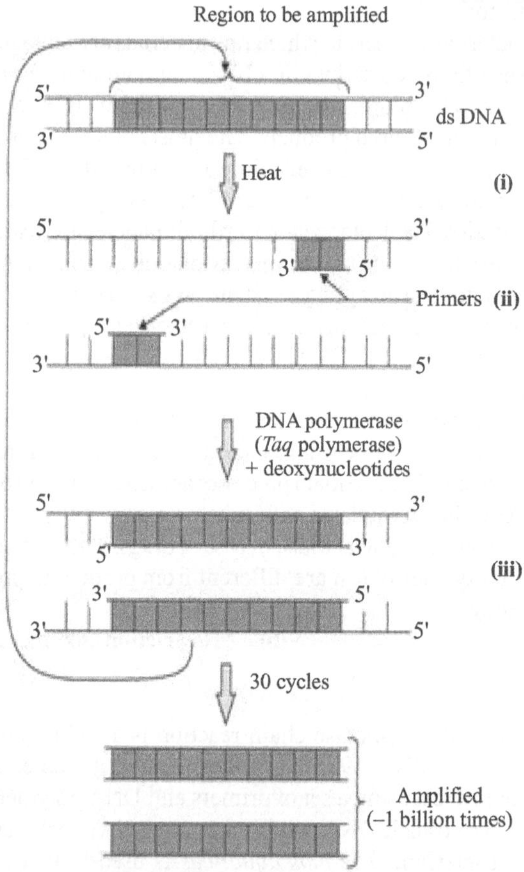

Fig.: Polymerase chain reaction

Note

- *PCR is based on the principle that a DNA molecule, when subjected to high temperature, splits into two strands due to denaturation.*
- *Applications of PCR: diagnosis of pathogens, diagnosis of specific mutations, DNA fingerprinting, in prenatal diagnosis and gene therapy.*

(b) **Restriction enzymes and DNA**

- Restriction enzymes are a class of nucleases present in bacteria responsible for restricting the growth of bacteriophages.
- They cut DNA molecules at a particular point by recognising a specific palindromic sequence of four to eight base pairs known as the recognition sequence. Once it finds its specific recognition sequence, it will bind to the DNA and cut each of the two strands of the double helix at specific points in their sugar-phosphate backbones.
- Restriction endonucleases are used in genetic engineering to form recombinant DNA molecules from different sources or genomes. When cut by the same restriction enzyme, the resultant DNA fragments have the same kind of sticky-ends and, these can be joined together (end-to-end) using DNA ligases. Thus, these are called molecular scissors.

Note

Hind II was the first restriction endonuclease to be discovered. Hind II always cuts DNA molecules at a particular point by recognising a specific sequence of six base pairs. This specific base sequence is called the recognition sequence for Hind II.

(c) **Chitinase**

- It is an enzyme used during DNA isolation from fungal cells.
- This enzyme acts on the chitin present in the cell wall of fungal cells and breaks them open to release DNA along with other macromolecules such as RNA, proteins, polysaccharides and also lipids.

12. Discuss with your teacher and find out how to distinguish between

(a) Plasmid DNA and Chromosomal DNA

(b) RNA and DNA

(c) Exonuclease and Endonuclease

Sol. (a) Difference between plasmid DNA and chromosomal DNA

S. No.	Plasmid DNA	Chromosomal DNA
1.	These are small, circular, extrachromosomal DNA molecules present freely in the cytoplasm of some organisms (bacteria and some fungi) in addition to large chromosomal DNA.	These are linear or circular, single- or double-stranded DNA molecules present in the nucleus, mitochondria and chloroplasts of eukaryotic cells and in the nucleoid region of prokaryotic cells.
2.	They replicate independent of chromosomal DNA.	They replicate when the cell divides.
3.	They are naked *i.e*., not associated with proteins.	They are associated with large proteins.
4.	They carry very few genes.	They carry large number of vital genes.
5.	Some plasmids confer advantage to their host such as resistance to antibiotics.	They carry out all the functions required for the growth, survival and reproduction of an organism.

(b) Difference between RNA and DNA

S. No.	RNA	DNA
1.	RNA or Ribonucleic acid is polymer of ribonucleotides.	DNA or Deoxyribonucleic acid is polymer of deoxyribonucleotides.
2.	It has ribose sugar.	It has deoxyribose sugar.
3.	It has adenine, guanine, cytosine and uracil as nitrogenous bases.	It has adenine, guanine, cytosine and thymine as nitrogenous bases.
4.	It is single-stranded molecule.	It is double-stranded molecule.
5.	Most of the RNA is present in cytoplasm with little amount inside the nucleus.	DNA is found in the nucleus, with a small amount in cell organelles such as mitochondria and chloroplast.
6.	It acts as genetic material in some retroviruses and transfers genetic code required for the synthesis of proteins from the nucleus to the ribosome.	It acts as genetic material in most of the organisms and stores genetic information.
7.	It is synthesised from DNA.	It is self replicating.

(c) Difference between exonuclease and endonuclease

S.No.	Exonuclease	Endonuclease
1.	Exonucleases are a type of nucleases that remove nucleotides in direction 5' → 3' or 3' → 5' from 5' or 3' ends respectively of one strand of double-stranded DNA or of single-stranded DNA.	Endonucleases are a type of nucleases that make cuts at specific positions within the DNA.
2.	They act on single strand of DNA or gaps in double stranded DNA.	They cleave one strand or both strands of double stranded DNA.
3.	They do not cut RNA. 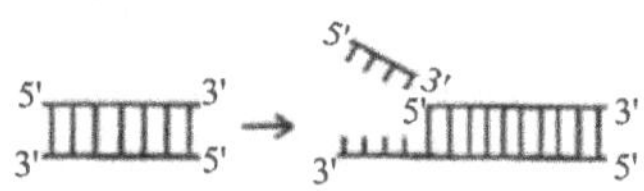	They may cut RNA. 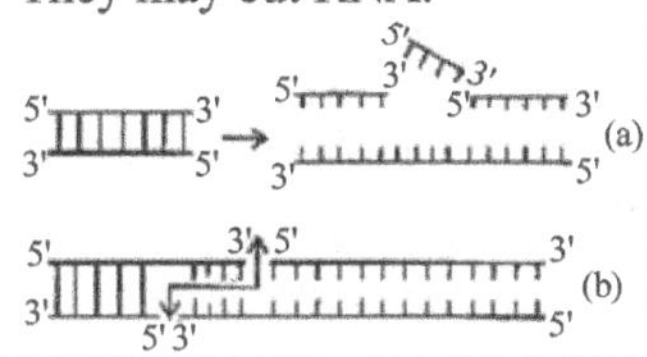

Chapter 12 BIOTECHNOLOGY AND ITS APPLICATIONS

CHAPTER AT A GLANCE

- The use of biology to develop technologies and products for the welfare of human beings is known as **biotechnology**.
- The applications of biotechnology include therapeutics, diagnostics, genetically modified crops for agriculture, processed food, bioremediation, waste treatment and energy production.

BIOTECHNOLOGICAL APPLICATION IN AGRICULTURE AND MEDICINE

- The use of biotechnology in agriculture is known as **green biotechnology**. The organisms formed after manipulation of genes is known as Genetically Modified Organisms such as crops, animals, plants, fungi, bacteria etc.
- **Genetic modifications** which have been introduced has :
  - made crops more tolerant to abiotic stresses [cold, drought, salt and heat].
  - reduced reliance on chemical pesticide (pest-resistant crop).
  - helped to reduce post harvest losses.
  - increased efficiency of mineral usage by plant to prevent early exhaustion of fertility of soil.
  - enhanced nutritional value of food, e.g., vitamin A enriched golden rice.
- **Genetically modified crops or transgenic crops** are prepared by transferring genes from one plant to other. The plant in which foreign genes are introduced are known as **transgenic crops**. These manipulations are done to introduce traits such as pest resistance, insect resistance, weed resistance etc.
- ***Bt*** **cotton is the first genetically modified crop** of the country. It is a pest resistant plant which resist attack of *Lepidopterans* insects. The plant *Bt* toxin gene cause death of insect larvae by causing cell lysis and swelling of epithelium of midgut.
- ***Bt*** **toxin** is biologically produced by bacterium called *Bacillus thuringiensis* (*Bt*).
- *Bt* toxin is coded by **gene** called **CRY genes**. These *Bt* toxin genes are isolated from bacteria and incorporated into several crop plants like cotton which has these lepidopteran insects as pests.
- *B. thuringiensis* forms protein crystals during a particular phase of their growth. These crystals contain a toxic **insecticidal protein**.

- The proteins encoded by the genes **cryIAc and cryIIAb control the cotton bollworms that of cryIAb control corn borer**.
- Pest resistant plant is a variety that is less susceptible to pest damage when compared with other crops.
- Prevention of nematode *Meloidegyne incognitia* parasitism on roots of tobacco plants is done by **(RNAi) – RNA interference technology.**
- RNAi is a **method of cellular defense in all eukaryotes**.
- RNAi is silencing of mRNA due to complementary double stranded RNA that prevents translation of mRNA [silencing]. It is used for nematode control in tobacco plant.
- Using *Agrobacterium* as a vector, nematode specific DNA is introduced into host plant which produces dsRNA. They initiate RNAi and silence specific mRNA when go inside nematode. Thus, parasite could not survive in transgenic host expressing specific dsRNA acting as **RNAi**.
- Tomato plant *Flavr savr* is genetically modified which produces much less cell wall degrading enzyme, **polygalactouronase**, responsible for fruit ripening. Therefore, the fruit of these plants have much larger and favourable shelf life.
- **Transgenic/genetically engineering plants** can also:
  - produce pharmaceutically important compounds such as human insulin, interferons, hormones, etc.
  - synthesise antibody and vaccines in fruits.
  - bear flowers with new colours and long life for better ornamental purposes.
- Insulin was extracted from pancreas of cattle, pigs in limited quantity.
- **Genetically - engineered insulin** helps in the management of diabetes after regular time intervals.
- Gene therapy is **alteration of specific genes** to modify the patient's genotype for the treatment of hereditary diseases like SCID, haemophilia and phenylketonuria.
- A gene cannot be directly inserted into a persons cell. It must be delivered to the cell using a carrier or vector. The vectors most commonly used in gene therapy are viruses.
- The **first clinical gene therapy** was given to 4 years old in 1990 with ADA deficiency.
- **Severely combined immuno deficiency disease (SCID)** patient has a defective gene for enzyme adenosine deaminase (ADA). Patient do not have T lymphocyte and don't mount immune response against pathogens. So to correct SCID with the help of **gene therapy:**
  - A WBC is extracted from bone marrow of sufferer and a good copy of human gene encoding ADA is introduced by **retrovirus** as vector.
  - This leads to WBC with a good copy of gene, in addition to existing faulty copy.

- The treated cells are reinjected to patient's bone marrow and cells play normal role in immune system.

- Genetics as well as infectious diseases can be diagnosed using probe consisting of short segment of dsDNA attached to fluorescent marker. These are used for identification of **food poisoning** (*Salmonella*), **pus forming** (*Staphylococcus*), **hepatitis virus, HIV of AIDS** using **ELISA**.
- ELISA is a laboratory test, which can quickly determine antigen or antibody levels in blood or other fluids.
- A single stranded DNA/RNA attached with radioactive molecule is called **molecular probe**. Molecular probes are used for detection of gene by complementary hybridising in cloned cell, followed by autoradiography.
- **Hirudin** is a protein that stops blood clotting. The gene encoding hirudin was chemically synthesised and then transferred into *Brassica napus*, where hirudin accumulates in seeds. The hirudin is purified and used as medicine.

TRANSGENIC ANIMALS AND ETHICAL ISSUES

- Animals that have their DNA manipulated to possess and express an extra (foreign) gene are known as **transgenic animals**. For example: rats, rabbits, pigs, sheep etc.
- Transgenic sheep produce clotting factor for haemophilics.
- Transgenic goat produce protein to dissolve clot, cure for coronary thrombosis.
- Transgenic cattle, sheep and fish grow most quickly and produce more meat.
- **Ethical issues** refer to the situation in which we need to select the best amongst the various alternatives. Same is the case with biotechnology as well.
- For reduction of **ethical issues** Indian government has set up organisation **GEAC [Genetic engineering approval committees]**, that make decision regarding validity of GM research and safety of introducing GMO in ecosystem.
- **Biopiracy** is unethical and illegal use of biodiversity resource of person concerned without any compensation.
- **Biopiracy of African super-sweet berries:** *Pentadiplandra brazzein* is a plant found in the west of South Africa. It is a vital source of protein known as **brazzein**.
- **Patent laws** are desirable not only to solve ethical issues related to GMO and introduction of new variety but also to prevent and flourish biodiversity and rich bioresource heritage of India.

EXERCISE

1. **Crystals of *Bt* toxin produced by some bacteria do not kill the bacteria themselves because –**
   (a) **bacteria are resistant to the toxin**
   (b) **toxin is immature**
   (c) **toxin is inactive**
   (d) **bacteria encloses toxin in a special sac.**

Sol. (c) Crystals of Bt toxin produced by some bacteria do not kill the bacteria themselves because toxin is present in inactive form. *Bt* toxin protein is produced by bacterium, *Bacillus thuringiensis*. It exists as inactive protoxins and is converted into an active form of toxin due to the alkaline pH of the gut of an insect upon ingestion.

2. **What are transgenic bacteria? Illustrate using any one example.**

Sol.
- *Transgenic bacteria* are those bacteria whose genome are manipulated by introduction of foreign gene from another organism using recombinant DNA technology. This introduced foreign gene is made to express in the host bacteria for the production of various commercially important products.
- *An example of transgenic bacteria* is *Escherichia coli* which produces synthetic human insulin. Two DNA sequences corresponding to A and B chains of human insulin are prepared and introduced in the plasmids. These recombinant plasmids are introduced into *E. coli*. This *E. coli* (now called transgenic) produces insulin chains A and B which are later extracted and combined by creating disulphide bonds to form human insulin.

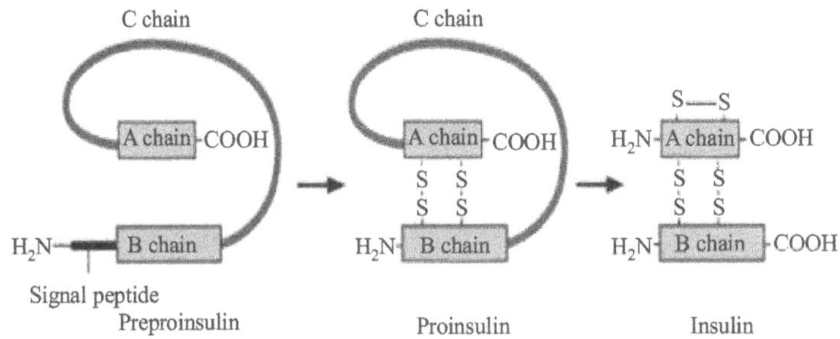

3. **Compare and contrast the advantages and disadvantages of production of genetically modified crops.**

Sol. Plants whose genes have been altered by manipulation are called genetically modified crops. GM crops have been advantageous in several ways and at the same time have some disadvantages also.

Contrast and comparison of advantages and disadvantages of genetically modified crops are as follows:

S. No.	Advantages	Disadvantages
1.	Most of the GM crops have been developed for pest resistance, which increases the crop productivity and therefore, reduces the reliance on chemical pesticides.	Pollens from pest resistant GM crops are harmful to beneficial insects such as larvae of monarch butterflies due to relatively similar physiology among insects. Also, crops share fields with other plants, including weeds. Gene flow from an herbicide-resistant crop into the weeds gives them a selective advantage leading to generation of superweeds.
2.	They are highly tolerant to unfavourable abiotic conditions (*cold*, *drought*, *salt*, *heat*).	Pollens of genetically modified crops will have the foreign gene. Cross pollination between GMO crops and non-GMO crops or wild relatives leading to spread of transgene to these plants (called genetic pollution) thereby decreasing their value for plant breeding programmes.
3.	Many varieties of GM food crops have been developed with enhanced nutritional quality. For example, golden rice is a transgenic variety of rice, which is rich in vitamin A.	Genetically modified crops produce proteins which were not present before. These novel proteins supply allergens and certain antibiotic resistance markers in the body and may trigger certain reactions such as allergies thus, affect human health. Antibiotic resistance marker gene may transfer from GM food to microflora in the gut of humans and animals or to the pathogens in the environment transforming them into strains that are resistant to antibiotic therapy. Nutritional composition of GM products may be affected in GM plants.

Contd. ...

4.	These plants prevent early exhaustion of fertility of soil by increasing their efficiency of mineral usage.	There is a risk associated with the cultivation of *Bt* crops due to contamination of soil by leaching of *Bt* toxin after harvest of *Bt* crops.

4. What are Cry proteins? Name an organism that produces it. How has man exploited this protein to his benefit?

Sol.
- *Cry proteins* are crystal proteins encoded by *cry genes*.
- These proteins are endotoxins produced by bacterium, *Bacillus thuringiensis* during a particular phase of their growth. *Bacillus thuringiensis* is a common Gram positive, spore-forming, soil bacterium.
- *Man has exploited Cry protein* for the production of insect-resistant transgenic *Bt* crops because this protein has insecticidal toxin which can kill specific insects such as lepidopterans (tobacco budworm, armyworm), coleopterans (beetles) and dipterans (flies, mosquitoes). Specific *Bt* toxin genes isolated from *Bacillus thuringiensis* are incorporated into the several crop plants such as cotton and corn. *Bt* toxin protein exists as inactive protoxin. When an insect ingests inactive toxin crystals, these are converted into active form of toxin due to the alkaline pH of the gut which solubilise the crystals. The activated toxin binds to the surface of midgut epithelial cells and creates pores that cause cell swelling and lysis and eventually cause death of the insect.

Note

When resources are limited, vegetative Bt cells undergo sporulation during which a spore is formed along with proteins accumulated in the cytoplasm of the cells as crystalline inclusions. Proteins in these crystals are called Cry (from Crystal). At the end of the sporulation process, crystals and spores are liberated concomitantly by lysis of the cells. Once Cry protein is ingested by a susceptible insect, the alkaline pH of its digestive tract denatures the insoluble crystals, making them soluble and thus amenable to being cut with proteases found in the insect gut, which liberate the cry toxin from the crystal. The Cry toxin is then inserted into the insect gut epithelial cell membrane, paralysing the digestive tract and forming a pore. The insect stops eating and starves to death; live Bt bacteria may also colonize the insect which can contribute to death.

5. What is gene therapy? Illustrate using the example of adenosine deaminase (ADA) deficiency.

Sol.
- *Gene therapy* is a collection of methods that uses genes to correct a gene defect diagnosed in a child or embryo. If a defective gene causes a necessary protein to be faulty or missing, gene therapy delivers a normal copy of the gene into the individual or embryo which restores the function of the protein by taking over the function of and compensating for the non-functional gene.

- The *first clinical gene therapy* was given in 1990 to a 4-year old girl with adenosine deaminase (ADA) deficiency. ADA deficiency causes SCID (Severe Combined Immuno Deficiency) in which B-lymphocytes and T-lymphocytes are not formed. The ADA gene provides instructions for producing the enzyme adenosine deaminase. This enzyme is produced in all cells, but the highest levels of adenosine deaminase occur in immune system cells called lymphocytes.

  In gene therapy for ADA deficiency,

  (i) Lymphocytes or bone marrow cells from the blood of the patient are grown in a culture outside the body.

  (ii) A functional ADA cDNA is then introduced into these lymphocytes or marrow cells using a retroviral vector.

  (iii) The transformed lymphocytes or marrow cells containing ADA gene are subsequently returned to the patient's bone marrow. Thus, the gene activated producing functional T-lymphocytes and activating the patients immune system.

Note

The adenosine deaminase (ADA) enzyme is important for the normal functioning of the immune system. The individual suffering from this disorder, arise due to deficiency of the ADA enzyme, can be cured by transplantation of bone marrow cells.

6. Digrammatically represent the experimental steps in cloning and expressing an human gene (say the gene for growth hormone) into a bacterium like *E. coli*?

Sol.
- DNA cloning, as the starting point for many genetic engineering approaches to biotechnology research, is a method of producing multiple identical copies of specific template DNA. It involves the use of a vector to carry the specific foreign DNA fragment into the host cell.
- The mechanism of cloning and transfer of gene for growth hormone into E.coli is represented below:

  Human growth hormone (hGH) is the naturally occurring growth hormone of humans or a genetically engineered form that is used to treat children with growth hormone deficiencies.

  Human growth hormone (hGH) is a small, single chain peptide hormone encoded by the GHN gene. It is produced by the anterior pituitary gland and is essential for normal growth and development in humans. The mature structure of hGH contains 191 amino acid residues. Since genes in eukaryotes are split genes with exons or coding sequences interrupted by introns or non-coding sequences, for the expression of gene for human growth hormone, cDNA synthesised from mRNA of human growth hormone is cloned through polymerase chain reaction (PCR). Cloned cDNA and vector are cut with the same restriction enzyme and both are ligated by using DNA ligase. The vector carrying cDNA is transformed into host, *E. coli* for expression. Transformed *E. coli* are cultured in growth medium for the expression of human growth hormone gene. The experimental steps in cloning and expression of gene for human growth hormone into a bacterium such as *E. coli* are as follows:

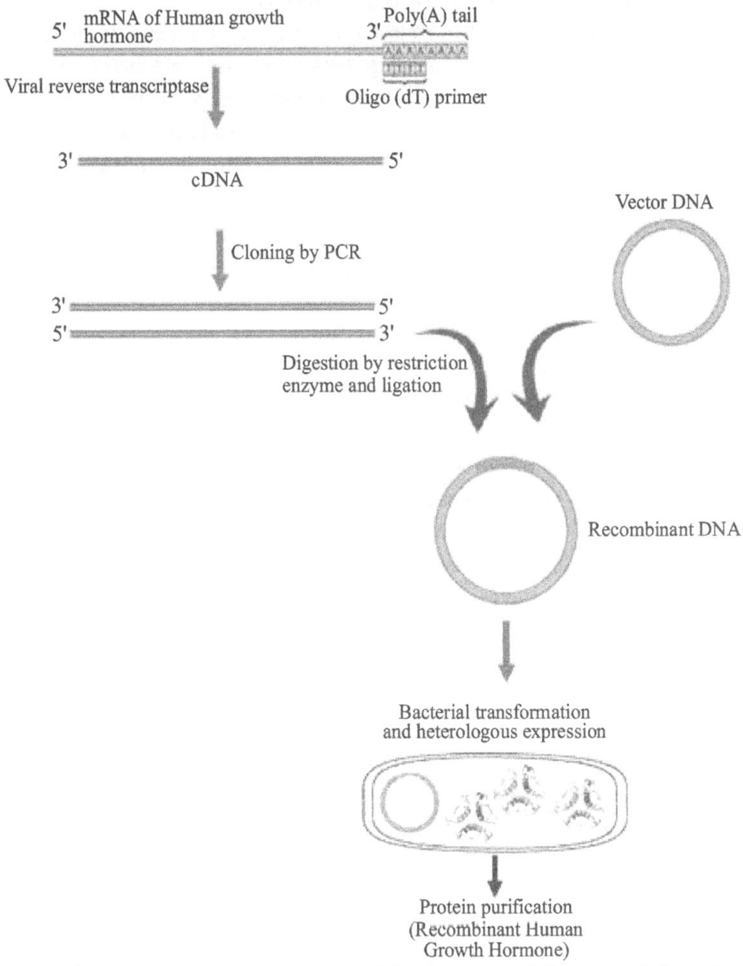

7. Can you suggest a method to remove oil (hydrocarbon) from seeds based on your understanding of rDNA technology and chemistry of oil?

Sol. Recombinant DNA technology (rDNA) is a technique used for manipulating the genetic material of an organism to obtain the desired result. The constituents of oil present in seed are glycerol and fatty acids.

The genes for the formation of glycerol or fatty acids which are the main constituents of oil, should be identified and removed from the seed by using enzyme restriction endonucleases. Such DNA molecule should then be treated with DNA ligases to join the broken ends. These cells when grown in a minimum nutrient medium, under aseptic conditions will differentiate into a new variety whose seeds will not have oil in them because the gene producing the oil has been removed.

8. Find out from internet what is golden rice.

Sol. Golden rice is a variety of rice (*Oryza sativa*) produced through recombinant DNA technology to biosynthesise beta-carotene, a precursor of vitamin A, in the edible parts of rice. It was developed by Ingo Potrykus from Swiss Federal Institute of Technology in Zurich, Switzerland and Peter Beyer from University of Freiburg in 1990. Golden Rice gets its name because the high levels of beta-carotene make it a golden-yellow colour. It was developed as a fortified food to be grown and consumed in areas where rice is a major staple food. It is generally consumed in its milled form in which outer layers (pericarp, tegmen and aleurone layers) are removed. The main reason for milling is to remove the oil-rich aleurone layer, which turns rancid upon storage. As a result, the edible part of rice grains consists of the endosperm, filled with starch granules and protein bodies, but it lacks several essential nutrients for the maintenance of health, such as carotenoids exhibiting provitamin A-activity. Thus, reliance on rice as a primary food staple leads to vitamin A deficiency (VAD). The deficiency of vitamin A causes childhood blindness in the developing world, and weakens the immune system, increasing vulnerability to illnesses such as measles, respiratory infections and diarrhoea, often leading to death.

9. Does our blood have proteases and nucleases?

Sol.
- Yes, protease and nuclease are found in blood.
- *Proteases* are enzymes that catalyse cleavage of peptide bonds in proteins.

  They are involved in many physiological reactions from digestion of proteins of food to highly regulated cascades. Proteases such as thrombin, factor XII (Hageman factor) and plasmin are found in blood serum and carry out functions such as blood coagulation, dissolution of blood clot and induction of physiological immune responses. Other proteases are found in leucocytes (elastase, cathepsin G) and play several different roles in metabolic control.
- *Nucleases* are enzymes that cleave phosphodiester bonds in nucleic acids. Some nucleases are DNA specific (DNase), some are RNA specific (RNase), and some degrade both DNA and RNA. Nucleases (such DNase and RNase) are also found in blood serum and lysosomes of white blood cells (macrophages) and help in degradation of DNA and RNA of pathogens and apoptotic cells.

Note

In blood, serum is the component that is neither a blood cell (serum does not contain white or red blood cells) nor a clotting factor. It is the blood plasma with the fibrinogen removed.

10. Consult internet and find out how to make orally active protein pharmaceutical. What is the major problem to be encountered?

Sol.

- *Orally active pharmaceutical proteins* are biologically active proteins or peptides which are adminisitered orally for the treatment of a variety of diseases, such as diabetes, cancer, infectious diseases, haemophilia, and anaemia. Common pharmaceutical proteins include antibodies, hormones, interleukins, enzymes and anticoagulants. Currently, most of all recombinant pharmaceutical proteins are produced in mammalian cells because mammalian cells are capable of producing high-quality proteins similar to the naturally occurring ones. In addition, many approved recombinant therapeutic proteins are generated in *Escherichia coli.*
- The *major problem encountered in oral delivery of proteins and peptides* is their degradation by proteolytic enzymes present in gastrointestinal tract, their poor stability in lower pH of gastric fluid, large molecular size and their inability to cross gastrointestinal membrane due to low lipophilicity. These characteristics lead to the low bioavailability of most orally administered peptides and short half-lives (<30 min) and failure of delivery of intact protein/peptide to the targeted site. Nano-carrier-based delivery is an appropriate choice of drug carriers owing to their property to protect proteins from degradation by the low pH conditions in stomach or by the proteolytic enzymes in the gastrointestinal tract.

13 Chapter ORGANISMS AND POPULATIONS

CHAPTER AT A GLANCE

- **Ecology** is a study of interactions between living organisms and its physical or abiotic or non-living environment.

ORGANISMS AND ITS ENVIRONMENT

- Organisms are the **basic unit of study in ecology**.
- Ecology is basically concerned with biological interactions at four levels. These levels are organism level, population level, community level and biome level.
- The **smallest level of organisation** is an **individual** of species and the largest level of organisation is **biosphere**.
- **Habitat** is a specific place or locality where an organism lives.
- The key elements that lead to so much variation in the conditions of different habitats can be subdivided into two components –
  - **Abiotic or nonliving or physical components** – Includes all the physical components, such as soil, temperature, water, light, etc.
  - **Biotic or living or biological components** – Includes all the living organisms.
- **Temperature** is the **most ecologically relevant environmental factor** ranging from below zero degree in polar regions and greater than 50°C at high altitudes in arid or deserts during summer.
- Majority of animals are cold-blooded or **poikilotherms or ectotherms** which do not have constant body temperature. Change in the temperature of environment affect mostly to poikilotherms. Eg. reptiles, fish and amphibians.
- Mammals and birds are **homeotherms** or warm-blooded animals with a constant body temperature irrespective of the environmental temperature.
- Many poikoilotherms undergoes an inactive phase, during winter season, called **hibernation**.
- Some animals also undergo a period of dormancy, called **aestivation**, during a drought or dry season.
- A few organisms, called **eurythermal**, can tolerate and thrive very well in a wide range of temperature. However, some organisms, are called **stenothermal**, and are restricted to a narrow range of temperature.

- Water is the most important factor influencing the life of organisms. It covers about 73% of Earth's surface.
- Aquatic organisms having wide range of salt tolerance are called **euryhaline**.
- Many freshwater animals cannot live for long in sea water and *vice versa* because of the osmotic problems, they would face.
- **Light is an important abiotic factor**. Life is not possible on earth without the presence of sun light.

  Plants produce food through photosynthesis, a process which is only possible when sunlight is available as a source of energy. Light is also essential for transpiration and flowering, and sometimes in germination of seeds.
- Light loving plants are known as **heliophytes** while shade loving plants are called **sciophytes**.
- **Soil** is the loose surface material consisting of inorganic particles and organic matter that covers most of the land surface.
- Soil provides the structural support & the source of water and nutrients for plants used in agriculture.
- Various characteristics of the soil such as soil composition, grain size and aggregation determine the percolation and water-holding capacity of the soil. These characteristics along with parameters such as pH, mineral composition and topography determine to a large extent the vegetation in many areas.
- The organism should try to maintain the constancy of its internal environment, a process called **homeostasis**, by monitoring changes in the external and internal environment.
- The term homeostasis was coined in 1930 by the physician **Walter Cannon**.
- **Biome** is a major complex biotic community which is characterized by distinctive plant and animal species and maintained under the climatic conditions of the region.
- The various possible ways the organisms cope up with the changing environment: regulate, conform, migrate, and suspend.
- Some organisms are able to maintain homeostasis by physiological (sometimes behavioural also) means which ensures constant body temperature, constant osmotic concentration, etc.
- About 99% of animals and nearly all plants cannot maintain a constant internal environment. Their body temperature changes with the temperature of the surrounding environment. In aquatic animals, the osmotic concentration of the body fluids changes with that of the osmotic concentration of water. These animals and plants are simply **conformers**.
- **Migrate** is a mechanism where the organism moves away temporarily from the stressful habitat to a more hospitable area and return when the conditions are favourable.
- **Suspend** is a mechanism employed by bacteria, fungi, lower plants and some animals to survive the unfavourable condition.

- Under unfavourable conditions many zooplankton species present in lakes and ponds, and certain insects are known to enter **diapause**, a stage of suspended development.
- **Adaptation** is any ability of an organism that enables an organism to survive and reproduce in its habitat.
- On the basis of various mode of adaptation plants are grouped as xerophytes (grow in dry habitat), hydrophytes (grow in water), heliophytes (growing in bright light), halophytes (growing in saline habitat), and sciophytes (growing in partial shades).

POPULATION AND ITS INTERACTION

- A population is a group of individuals of the same species within a community. It can also be defined as the total number of species of other class of organisms in a defined area or habitat.
- **Population growth** refers to change in the size of a population-which can be either positive or negative-over time, depending on the balance of births and deaths. If there are many deaths, the world's population will grow very slowly or can even decline. Population growth is measured in both absolute and relative terms.
- The nature of population is determined by various factors such as **density, birth rate or natality, death rate or mortality, emigration, immigration and sex ratio**.
- There are mainly **two types of population growth curves** – J-shaped or exponential growth curve, and S-shaped or logistic growth curve.
- J-shaped growth curve is a curve on a graph that records the situation in which, in a new environment, the population density of an organism increases rapidly in an exponential or logarithmic form, but then stops abruptly as environmental resistance or some other factors suddenly becomes effective.
- **S-shaped or logistic growth curve** is type of growth curve is shown by the yeast growth under laboratory conditions.
- The S-shape (sigmoid) curve is generated when a population approaches the environment's carrying capacity.
- It has five phases –
  - (i) Lag phase
  - (ii) Positive acceleration phase
  - (iii) Exponential phase
  - (iv) Negative acceleration phase
  - (v) Stationary phase

Population Interaction

- Some species of insects and frogs are cryptically-coloured to avoid being detected easily by the predator. This is called **camouflage**.
- **Amensalism** is a relationship in which one species is harmed whereas the other is unaffected.

- **Competition** is defined as a process in which the fitness of one species is significantly lower in the presence of another species.
- Competition is of two types – intraspecific (between individuals of same species) & inter specific (between individuals of different species).
- **Parasitism** is a relationship between two species in which one benefits on the host (harm) of the other. It is always an one side relationship for the parasite which is always benefitted from the host.
- The interaction in which one species benefits and the other is neither harmed nor benefited is known as **commensalism.**
  - The **examples showing commensalism are** orchids which grow as epiphytes on mango or other fruit trees.
  - Orchids are benefited by getting a shelter, while the tree is neither benefited nor harmed.
- **Mutualism** interaction is a positive reciprocal relationship between two different species.
  - It confers benefits on both the interacting species.
  - For examples : **Lichens** represent an intimate mutualistic relationship between a fungus and green algae.
- **Predation** is an interaction between members in which one population adversely affects the other by direct attack (capture, kill and eat) but is nevertheless dependent on other. The former is called **predators** & the latter is called **prey.**
- Predation also help in maintaining species diversity in a community, by reducing the intensity of competition among competing prey species.
- **Biological control** is a method of reducing or eliminating plant pests by introducing predators or micro-organisms that attack the targeted pests but spare other species in the area.

EXERCISE

1. How is diapause different from hibernation?

Sol.

S. No.	Diapause	Hibernation
1.	It is a stage of suspended development under unfavourable conditions. It is a special type of aestivation.	Also called winter sleep, it is a resting stage where in animals slow down their metabolism and remain inactive to escape winters by hiding themselves in their shelters.
2.	It is exhibited by many zooplankton species in lakes and ponds during their development.	It is exhibited by bats, squirrels, and other rodents.

2. If a marine fish is placed in a fresh water aquarium, will the fish be able to survive? Why or why not?

Sol. Seawater or marine fish have evolved osmoregulatory mechanisms that permit them to excrete excess salts in a hypertonic environment. Since the salt content in their blood is much lower than that of seawater, they constantly tend to lose water and build up salt. To replace the water loss, they continually drink seawater. Since their small kidney can only excrete relatively small amount of urine, the excretion of salt additionally takes place in the gills where chloride cells secreted excess sodium and chloride ions out into the sea.

If marine fish is placed in a fresh water aquarium, it will not be able to survive as they are not able to regulate water entering its body. The body of a marine fish has high salt concentration to surrounding fresh water so water enters the fish's body due to osmosis. Without any active regulation of this process, fishes would swell and get bigger and bigger leading to its death.

In order to survive in freshwater, marine fish must not drink much water and its kidneys must produce a large amount of urine, leading to loss of salts. In order to maintain a sufficient salt level, chloride cells in the gills must take up ions from the water. But osmoregulation of marine fish works in reverse direction, so it will not be able to survive in opposite environment.

Note

Body of marine fish are adapted to high salt concentrations of the marine environment. Therefore, the body fluid concentration of marine fish is much higher than that of fresh water.

3. Most living organisms cannot survive at temperature above 45°C. How are some microbes able to live in habitats with temperatures exceeding 100°C?

Sol. In most living organisms, the metabolic reactions and hence all the physiological functions proceed optimally in a narrow temperature range such as in humans, it is 37°C. Thus, they cannot survive at temperatures above 45°C as high temperature causes denaturation of their enzymes.

Some microbes such as archaebacteria *flourish in hot springs and deep sea hydrothermal vents where temperatures far exceed 100°C*. Because:

(i) They have thermostable enzymes which can perform their catalytic reactions even at high temperatures, without being denatured.

(ii) Some archaea have membranes with more stable components called glycerol-ether lipids which help them to survive in extreme environments.

(iii) These microbes avoid DNA denaturation at high temperature by proteins such as type I topoisomerase that catalyses positive supercoiling of closed circular DNA. Positively supercoiled DNA appears to resist degradation more than negatively supercoiled DNA.

Note

Thermophilic proteins have several adaptations that give the protein the ability to retain structure and function in extremes of temperature. Some of the most prominent are increased number of large hydrophobic residues, disulfide bonds, and ionic interactions.

4. List the attributes that populations but not individuals possess.

Sol. Population is a group of individuals of same species living in a well defined geographical area, sharing or competing for similar resources and potentially interbreeding. A population has certain attributes whereas, an individual organism does not.

The *list of attributes possessed by population but not by an individual are as follows*:

(i) *Natality or Birth rate*: It is the ratio of the number of births occurring in a population in a given period to the size of the population.

(ii) *Mortality or Death rate*: It is the ratio of the number of deaths occurring in a population in a given period to the size of the population.

(iii) *Sex ratio*: It is the ratio of males to females in a population.

(iv) *Population age distribution*: It refers to the proportionate number of individuals in successive age categories in a given population.

(v) *Population density*: It is the number of organisms that make up a population in a defined area.

5. If a population growing exponentially double in size in 3 years, what is the intrinsic rate of increase (r) of the population?

Sol. The population growth is exponential when resources are unlimited. The intrinsic rate of increase (r) can be calculated by exponential growth equation which is:

$N_t = N_O e^{rt}$

where, N_t = population density after time t

N_o = population density at time zero

r = intrinsic rate of natural increase

e = the base of natural logarithms

Given

$N_o = x$

$N_t = 2x$

$t = 3$ years

From equation,

$N_t = N_o e^{rt}$

$2x = x e^{3r}$

$\Rightarrow \quad 2 = e^{3r}$

Taking L_n b/s, we get,

$$\ell_n 2 = \ell_n e^{3r}$$

$$\Rightarrow \ell_n 2 = 3r\, \ell_n e \qquad (\because \ell_n ab = b\ell_n a)$$

$$\Rightarrow \ell_n 2 = 3r \qquad (\because \ell_n e = 1)$$

$$\Rightarrow r = \frac{\ell_n 2}{3}$$

$$r = \frac{2.303 \log 2}{3} \qquad (\because \ell_n a = 2.303 \log a)$$

$$r = \frac{2.303 \times 0.301}{3} \qquad (\because \log 2 = 0.301)$$

$$r = 0.231$$

$\therefore$ Intrinsic rate of natural increase of population $= r \times 100\%$
$= 0.231 \times 100\% = 23.1\%$

7. Name important defence mechanisms in plants against herbivory.

Sol. Herbivores are the predators of plants. Herbivory is the act of eating plants or plant like organisms. This problem is severe for plants because they cannot run away from their predators.

So as to counter the attack of herbivores, plants have *evolved diverse morphological and chemical defenses.*

(i) *Morphological defenses*: These defenses include development of some morphological structures or changes that provide mechanical protection on the surface of the plants. Examples of morphological defenses are:
- Plants develop spiny-structures like spines, thorns and prickles which discourage animals by causing physical damage or by inducing rashes and allergic reactions. Thorns in *Acacia* and cactus are the most common morphological means of defense.
- Trichomes are hair-like outgrowths from the epidermis of stem, leaves, and even fruits, and occur in several forms such as straight, spiral, stellate, hooked, and glandular to defend the plants against many insects.
- In some plant leaves hardened to provide defense to plants against herbivores by reducing the palatability and digestibility of the tissues.

(ii) *Chemical defences*: The chemical defenses involve toxic compounds which are produced constitutively or in response to plant damage, and affect feeding, growth, reproduction and survival of herbivores. Examples of such defenses are:
- *Calotropis* produces highly poisonous cardiac glycosides that is why any cattle or goats do not browse on this plant.

- Volatile oils produced by mint and sage discourage predators with noxious odours.
- Quinine prevent herbivory by its repellent tastes.
- Other alkaloids such as caffeine and opioids affect herbivores by causing excessive stimulation and lethargy respectively.
- Some compounds become toxic after ingestion such as glycol cyanide in the cassava root releases cyanide only upon ingestion by the herbivore.
- Foxgloves produce several deadly chemicals, namely cardiac and steroidal glycosides which on ingestion cause nausea, vomiting, hallucinations, convulsions, or death.
- Other chemical substances that are produced by plants as defenses against grazers and browsers are nicotine, caffeine, quinine, strychnine, opium, etc.

7. **An orchid plant is growing on the branch of mango tree. How do you describe this interaction between the orchid and the mango tree?**

Sol. An orchid is an epiphyte that grows on the branches of other plants such as mango for physical support. Most epiphytes live in tropical or temperate rainforests, where humidity and competition for sunlight are high. Thus, by growing on the branches of high plants, orchids are elevated and receive more sunlight and get protection from herbivores. In this interaction, only orchid is benefitted whereas mango is neither harmed nor benefitted. So, this interaction between orchid and mango is an example of commensalism.

8. **What is the ecological principle behind the biological control method of managing with pest insects?**

Sol. Biological control is to keep pest populations below damaging levels by using other living organisms which are their natural enemies e.g., use of ladybird and dragonflies to get rid of aphids and mosquitoes, respectively. The *ecological principle behind the biological control method adopted in agriculture to manage pest insects* is based on the natural mechanism called predation.

Note

Predation is a biological interaction between the predator and the prey, whereby the predator feeds on the prey. Hence, the predators regulate the population of preys in a habitat, thereby helping in the management of pest insects.

9. **Distinguish between the following:**
   (a) **Hibernation and Aestivation**
   (b) **Ectotherm and endotherm**

Sol. (a) Difference between hibernation and aestivation

S. No.	Hibernation	Aestivation
1.	It is winter sleep in which an animal passes the winter period in dormant condition.	It is winter sleep in which animal passes the summer period to avoid heat and desiccation in dormant condition.
2.	Hibernating animal rests in the warm place.	Aestivating animal rests in cool or shady and moist place.
3.	Animals that hibernate include insects, birds and mammals.	Animals that aestivate include many reptiles and amphibians such as desert tortoises, crocodiles, and salamanders.

(b) Difference between ectotherms and endotherms

S. No.	Ectotherms	Endotherms
1.	Ectotherms are those animals that do not have the ability to produce sufficient internal metabolic heat to maintain a constant body temperature.	Endotherms are animals which can generate heat within their body to maintain a constant body temperature independently of the environmental temperature.
2.	All animals except mammals and birds are ectotherms, and are often described as poikilotherms cold-blooded animals.	Mammals and birds are endotherms and are often described as homeotherms or warm-blooded animals.

10. Write a short note on

(a) Adaptations of desert plants and animals

(b) Adaptations of plants to water scarcity

(c) Behavioural adaptations in animals

(d) Importance of light to plants

(e) Effect of temperature or water scarcity and the adaptations of animals.

Sol. (a) Adaptations of desert plants and animals

- The *adaptations that allow plants* to minimise water loss in high temperature and water scarce conditions of desert plants are as follows:
  - (i) Presence of thick cuticle on their leaf surfaces.
  - (ii) Arrangement of stomata in deep pits (sunken) to minimise water loss through transpiration.
  - (iii) Presence of special photosynthetic pathway (CAM) that enables their stomata to remain closed during day time.
  - (iv) Reduction of leaves into spines and photosynthesis by the flattened stems in some desert plants like *Opuntia.*

- The *adaptations in desert animals* that help to acquire and retain water and also to regulate temperature thereby making their survival possible in the harsh conditions of the desert are as follows:
  - (i) Avoid being out in the sun during the hottest part of the day by either staying in their burrows as in most animals or sleeping during the daytime in their burrows or dens and hunting only during the night when the temperatures drop as in nocturnals.
  - (ii) Ability to concentrate urine so as to use minimal volume of water to remove excretory products.
  - (iii) Meeting the water requirements from water produced as byproduct through internal fat oxidation in the absence of an external source of water such as in the kangaroo rat .
  - (iv) Excreting concentrated urine and solid faeces.
  - (v) Possessing long body parts that provide greater body surface to dissipate heat.

(b) Adaptations of plants to water scarcity

- Plants have evolved following adaptations to survive under conditions of water scarcity by minimising water loss and optimisation of water uptake:
  - (i) They develop deep root system to reach underground water.
  - (ii) They bear thick cuticles and sunken stomata on the surface of their leaves to reduce transpiration.
  - (iii) They store water in their flesh stem and leaves.
  - (iv) Plants often shed leaves during dry periods and enter into a state of deep dormancy.
  - (v) Higher plants produce seeds and some other vegetative reproductive structures as means to tide over periods of stress.
- These structures remain in the state of dormancy during unfavourable conditions and germinate to form new plants under favourable moisture and temperature conditions.

(c) Behavioural adaptations in animals

- Animals *show following behavioural adaptations* to cope up with variations in their environment:
  - (i) Some animals move away temporarily from the stressful habitat to a more hospitable area and return when stressful period is over. For example, many animals, particularly birds, during winter undertake long-distance migrations to more hospitable areas.
  - (ii) Animals may avoid the stress by escaping in time through hibernation as in bears during winter or by aestivation as in snails and fish to avoid heat and desiccation.
  - (iii) Some organisms such as desert lizards bask in the sun and absorb heat when their body temperature drops below the comfort zone, but move into shade when the ambient temperature starts increasing.

(iv) Some animals make burrows into the soil to hide and escape from the above-ground heat.

(d) Importance of light to plants

- Light affects plants through three different aspects, *i.e.*, quantity, quality and duration.
- It is *important for following aspects of growth and development in plants*:
  (i) Plants use light as a source of energy for photosynthesis.
  (ii) Light is required for chlorophyll formation in many higher plants.
  (iii) Plant leaf stomatal opening is controlled by light. Both red and blue light stimulate stomatal opening.
  (iv) Light is responsible for transpiration which is responsible for absorption of water and pulling of water column in the upward direction (ascent of sap).
  (v) Sunlight is also required by the plants to meet their photoperiodic requirement for flowering.

(e) Effect of temperature or water scarcity on adaptations of animals:

- *Effect of temperature*
  (i) Temperature plays an important role in maintaining the role of enzymes, its metabolism, activity and other physiological functions. It also affects the habitat, geographical distribution and pigmentation.
  (ii) The animals of the cold regions develop thick fur and have more fat so as to avoid the cold conditions.
  (iii) Certain animals which cannot regulate the temperature for e.g. desserts lizards bask in the sun to absorb heat and move to shade when the temperature increases.
  (iv) Animals also avoid cold conditions by migration or hibernation.
- *Animals tend to adapt to the water scarcity by*
  (i) Excreting solid urine and faeces.
  (ii) Having spiny skin and highly cornified skin
  (iii) Changing the feeding habits. For this they come out during the night or early morning for feeding purposes to prevent loss of water.

11. List the various abiotic environmental factors.

Sol. *Various abiotic environmental factors* are:

(i) *Temperature*: It is the most important environmental factor. It affects the kinetics of enzymes and through it the metabolic activity and other physiological functions of the organism. The levels of thermal tolerance of different species determine to a large extent their geographical distribution.

(ii) *Water*: It is another most important factor influencing the life of organisms. Life is unsustainable without water. The productivity and distribution of plants is also heavily dependent on water. For aquatic organisms, the quality (chemical composition, pH) of water becomes important.

(iii) *Light*: Photosynthesis, a process through which all living organisms get their food, is only possible when sunlight is available as a source of energy. Many plants are also dependent on sunlight to meet their photoperiodic requirement for flowering. It is important for many animals also. Animals use the diurnal and seasonal variations in light intensity and duration (photoperiod) as cues for timing their foraging, reproductive and migratory activities. The spectral quality of solar radiation is also important for life.

(iv) *Soil*: The nature and properties of soil which varies in different places, is dependent on the climate, the weathering process, whether soil is transported or sedimentary and how soil development occurred. Various characteristics of the soil such as soil composition, grain size and aggregation determine the percolation and water holding capacity of the soils. These characteristics along with parameters such as pH, mineral composition and topography determine to a large extent the vegetation in any area. This in turn dictates the type of animals that can be supported.

12. Give an example for:

(a) An endothermic animal

(b) An ectothermic animal

(c) An organism of benthic zone

Sol. (a) *Endothermic animals* generate their body heat to maintain a constant body temperature independent of environment, e.g., humans (mammals).

(b) *Exothermic animals* cannot maintain a constant internal environment and their body temperature changes with the changes in the external environment, e.g., fish, amphibians and reptiles.

(c) *Benthic animals* live at the bottom of water body such as a lake or ocean, e.g., sea anemone.

13. Define population and community.

Sol. *Population* is a group of individuals of same species living in a well defined geographical area, share or compete for similar resources, potentially interbreed, e.g., cormorants (aquatic birds) in a wetland, rats in an abandoned dwelling, teakwood trees in a forest tract, bacteria in a culture plate and lotus plants in a pond.

Community is a group or association of populations of two or more different species that occupy the same geographical area and interact with each other, e.g., a population of mallard ducks, and a population of cattail (*Typha Latifolia*) plants in a freshwater pond.

14. Define the following terms and give one example for each:
(a) Commensalism (b) Parasitism
(c) Camouflage (d) Mutualism
(e) Interspecific competition

Sol. (a) Commensalism

- It is a interspecific positive interaction in which, one species is benefitted and the other is neither harmed nor benefitted.
- The *examples of commensalism* are barnacles growing on the back of a whale, the cattle egret forging close to grazing cattle and clown fish living among sea anemone. In these examples, barnacles, cattle egret and clown fish are the organisms that are benefitted whereas whale, cattle and sea anemone do not get any benefit.

(b) Parasitism

- It is an interaction between two species in which one organism called parasite) lives on or within the other organism called the host for food or shelter.
- Parasites harm the host and may reduce the survival, growth and reproduction of the host eventually its population density. So, in this interaction, one organism is benefited and the other is harmed.
- Example: ticks on dogs, *Plasmodium* feeding upon liver cells and RBCs of man.

(c) Camouflage

- It is an adaptation in animals that allows them to blend in with their surroundings. This strategy helps prey to avoid being detected easily by the predator and helps predator to ambush their prey.
- Example, stone fish always sit perfectly still, on the sea floor, in their preferred habitat of coral and rocky reefs and looks like an encrusted rock or lump of coral. This helps them remain unnoticed by its prey.

(d) Mutualism

- In this interaction, both the interacting organisms in the association are benefitted.
- The examples of are lichens (mutualistic relationship between a fungus and photosynthesising algae or cyanobacteria), mycorrhizae (association between fungi and the roots of higher plants) and association between plants and their pollinators.

(e) Interspecific competition

- It is a form of competition in which individuals of different species compete for the same resources in an ecosystem. It is a type of antagonistic interaction.
- Example, competition between flamingos and fishes for their common food, the zooplankton in the lake.

15. With the help of suitable diagram describe the logistic population growth curve.

Sol. When resources are unlimited, populations exhibit exponential growth, resulting in a J-shaped curve, which is not the case in the real world. In nature, a given habitat has enough resources to support a maximum possible number, beyond which no further growth is possible. This population size, which represents the maximum population size that a particular environment can support, is called the carrying capacity, or K.

When resources are limited, populations exhibit logistic growth. In such a growth, a population initially show a lag phase, followed by phases of acceleration and deceleration and finally an asymptote, when the population density reaches the carrying capacity resulting in an S-shaped curve. This type of population growth is called *Verhulst-Pearl Logistic Growth* and is described by the following equation:

$$dN/dt = rN[K - N/K]$$

Where, r = intrinsic rate of natural increase
N = population density at time t
K = carrying capacity

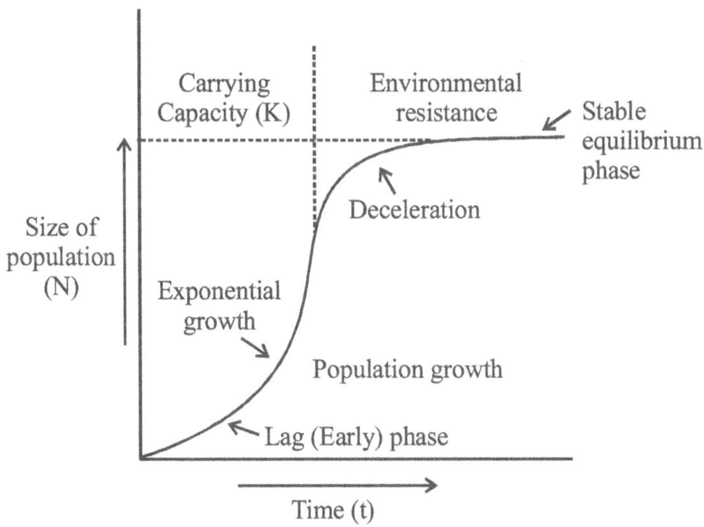

Fig. : Logistic population growth curve or S-shaped curve

16. Select the statement which explains best parasitism.

(a) One organism is benefited.

(b) Both the organisms are benefited.

(c) One organism is benefited, other is not affected.

(d) One organism is benefited, other is affected.

Sol. **(d)** Parasitism is a relationship between species, where one organism called the parasite lives on or in another organism called the host for food and/or shelter. Parasite causes some harm to its host, and is adapted structurally to this way of life. So, in such a relationship, parasite is benefited and the host is harmed.

For example, ticks and lice (parasites) present on the human body represent this interaction where in the parasites receive benefit (as they derive nourishment by feeding on the blood of humans). On the other hand, these parasites reduce host fitness and cause harm to the human body.

17. List any three important characteristics of a population and explain.

Sol. The *three important characteristics of a population* are :

(i) **Population density :** It refers to the number of organisms that make up a population in a defined area.

(ii) **Natality or Birth rate :** The birth rate is determined by the number of individuals that are added to a given population during a given period of time.

(iii) **Mortality or Death rate :** The death rate or mortality represents a decrease in a given population due to deaths during a given period of time. Generally, the death of individuals in a population is expressed by specific mortality which is described as the mortality for given age group.

Chapter 14

ECOSYSTEM

CHAPTER AT A GLANCE

- **Ecosystem** is the functional unit of nature where living organisms interact with each other and with their environment.
- Ecosystem can be recognised as self regulating and self sustaining units of landscapes that may be *terrestrial* or *aquatic*.
- Forests, grasslands and deserts are **examples of terrestrial ecosystems**. The aquatic ecosystems can be either fresh water (ponds, lakes, streams) or salt water (marine estuaries) type.
- Ecosystem may be **natural** (forest, sea); if developed under natural conditions or **artificial** (garden, agriculture) if created by man.

COMPONENTS OF ECOSYSTEM

- An ecosystem has **two basic components–abiotic (non-living)** and **biotic (living organisms)**.
- There are **three biotic components** : producers, consumers and decomposers. Abiotic components may be –
  - **Physical or climatic components,** like temperature, water, light, etc.
  - **Inorganic compounds :** Like water, minerals (sulphur, nitrogen, phosphorus etc.) and atmospheric gases (O_2, CO_2, N_2, etc.)
  - **Organic compounds :** These includes the organic substances present in the dead bodies of plants and animals. e.g., proteins, carbohydrates liquids etc.
- The proper functioning of an ecosystem takes place through the following processes :
  - Productivity
  - Decomposition
  - Relationship of producers and consumers,
  - Flow of energy through different trophic levels,
  - Cycling of nutrients.
- **Standing crop** is the amount of living biomass in an ecosystem. It indicates the productivity & luxuriance of growth.
- The amount of nutrients, e.g., nitrogen, phosphorus & calcium present in the soil at any given time is known as **standing state**.

PRODUCTIVITY

- The rate of biomass production is called **productivity**. It is of **two types** – primary productivity and secondary productivity.
- **Primary productivity** is the amount of biomass produced per unit area over a time period by plants during photosynthesis.It is expressed in terms of weight (g^{-2}) or energy (kcal m^{-2}). It is of two types:
  (i) **Gross Primary Productivity (GPP)** – It is the rate of production of biomass or accumulation of energy by green plants per unit area per unit time.
  (ii) **Net Primary Productivity (NPP)** – It is the amount of biomass which has been stored by green plants.
  Net primary productivity = Gross primary productivity – Respiration losses.
  (or GPP–R = NPP)
- **Secondary productivity** is the amount of biomass synthesised by consumers per unit area per unit time.

DECOMPOSITION

- **Decomposition** is the breakdown of complex organic compounds of dead bodies of plants and animals into simpler inorganic compounds like CO_2, water & various nutrients.
- The various processes involved in decomposition are **fragmentation, leaching, catabolism, humification, and mineralisation**.
- The organisms carrying out decomposition are called **decomposers**.
- Decomposers include **micro-organisms** (bacteria and fungi), **detritivores** (earthworm) and some parasites.

ENERGY FLOW

- The rate of energy transfer between elements of an ecological system is called **energy flow**.
- **Sun is the ultimate source of energy** for all the organisms of an ecosystem. 50% of the total solar radiation that falls on earth is **Photosynthetically Active Radiation (PAR)**.
- The flow of energy in an ecosystem is **unidirectional**. That is, it flows from the producer level to the consumer level and never in the reverse direction. Hence energy can be used only once in the ecosystem.
- **Only about 10% of the biomass is transferred from one** trophic level to the next one is a food chain. And only about 10% of chemical energy is retained at each trophic level. This is called **10% law of Lindeman (1942)**.
- **Producers** include green plants which are capable of manufacturing their own food. These are able to fix the energy obtained from the sun.

- **Consumers (phagotrophs)** cannot make their own food but are directly or indirectly dependent on producers for obtaining food.
- Consumers may be :
  - Primary consumers or **herbivores**.
  - Secondary consumers or **primary carnivores**.
  - Tertiary consumers or **secondary carnivores**.
  - Quartenery consumers.
- Primary consumers obtain their food by directly feeding on producers (plants), secondary consumers from primary consumers (herbivores) and tertiary consumers from secondary consumers.

Food Chain and Food Web

- **Food chain** is an order or sequence of different organisms which are arranged in a way that the food is passed from one type of organism to other organisms such that the organisms of one order or trophic level are the food of the organisms of next order.
  - **Grazing food chain** – Begins with plants and ends in carnivores. Eg. Grass → Grasshopper → Lizard → Hawk.
  - **Detritus food chain** – Begins with dead organic matter and made up of decomposers.
- **Food web** refers to a group of inter- related food chains in a particular community. Under natural conditions, the linear arrangement of food chain hardly occurs & these remain indeed inter-connected with each other through different types of organisms at different trophic level.

ECOLOGICAL PYRAMID

- The number of individuals present or amount of biomass synthesised or amount of energy stored at successive trophic levels in an ecosystem can be graphically represented in the form of pyramids. These are called **ecological or Eltonian pyramids.**
- Three ecological pyramids which are studied are – pyramid of number, pyramid of biomass and pyramid of energy.
  - Pyramid of number is usually upright.
  - The pyramid of number of a single tree is **spindle-shaped**.
  - Pyramid of biomass of terrestial ecosystem is **upright** because at each successive trophic level the biomass tends to decrease, starting from primary producers and ending in top consumers.
  - Pyramid of biomass of aquatic ecosystem is inverted.
  - Pyramid of energy is always **upright** because during the flow of energy from one trophic level to the next one, there always occurs a loss of energy.

BIOGEOCHEMICAL CYCLES

- Cyclic events by which various nutrients which are essential for the living organisms are transferred from one form to other. During these cycles, the nutrients pass from the biotic components to the abiotic components and vice-versa,; hence these are also called **biogeochemical cycles. Two types of nutrient cycles** are –
  - (i) **Gaseous cycles** (nitrogen, carbon cycles)
  - (ii) **Sedimentary cycles** (phosphorus, sulphur cycles)

Carbon cycle

- Carbon is present as CO_2 in atmosphere, as graphite and carbonates in rocks and also in fossil fuels (coal, petroleum).
- Ocean are big reservoirs of carbon.
- The cyclic representation of carbon assimilation by green plants (photosynthesis) which then passes into bodies of animals (plants are eaten) and finally during respiration of plants & animals & decompositions by microbes, the carbon dioxide is returned back to the atmosphere. Thus carbon is cycled through transfer and transformation between biotic and abiotic components.

Phosphorus cycle

- Phosphorus is present in
  - biomembranes (as phospholipids)
  - nucleic acids (as phosphoric acid)
  - nucleotides (as AMP, ADP, ATP etc.)
  - bones and teeth (as hydroxyapetite)
- Phosphorus is released during the decomposition of plant and animal remains.
- The released phosphorus may reach the deeper layers of soil and gets deposited as phosphate rocks.
- Phosphorus containing rocks are mined for manufacture of fertilisers, which provide an additional supply of an organic phosphates to the abiotic environment.

EXERCISE

1. **Fill in the blanks.**
   - **(a) Plants are called as_______because they fix carbon dioxide.**
   - **(b) In an ecosystem dominated by trees, the pyramid (of numbers) is_______type.**
   - **(c) In aquatic ecosystems, the limiting factor for the productivity is______.**
   - **(d) Common detritivores in our ecosystem are_______.**
   - **(e) The major reservoir of carbon on earth is______.**

Sol. (a) autotrophs (or producers)
(b) inverted
(c) sunlight
(d) earthworm, bacteria and fungi
(e) oceans

2. Which one of the following has the largest population in a food chain?
(a) Producers **(b) Primary consumers**
(c) Secondary consumers **(d) Decomposers**

Sol. (d) Decomposers are those organisms, especially a soil bacterium, fungus, or invertebrate that decomposes organic material. They form the largest population in a food chain because they are present at the top trophic level of the food chain and break down dead organic material to water, carbon dioxide, minerals and other simple chemicals which can again be consumed by green plants. Dead organic material occurs in form of leaf litter, dead wood, animal carcasses and faeces.

Note

If decomposers weren't in the ecosystem, the plants would not get essential nutrients, and dead matter and waste would pile up.

3. The second trophic level in a lake is:
(a) Phytoplankton **(b) Zooplankton**
(c) Benthos **(d) Fishes**

Sol. (b) Primary producers such as phytoplankton and algae form the lowest trophic level of food chain in a lake. These primary producers are eaten by primary consumers such as zooplanktons. Primary consumers occupy the second trophic level and are eaten by secondary consumers such as small fish. Tertiary consumers such as large fish eat the secondary consumers and are eaten by top level predators which include fish-eating birds.

4. Secondary producers are:
(a) Herbivores **(b) Producers**
(c) Carnivores **(d) None of these**

Sol. (a) A secondary producer is a herbivore, an animal that eats plant matter and, in turn, is food for a predator. Although herbivores are consumers, they are a source of food for carnivores. Since they eat plants, they are eating the primary producers, making them primary consumers. But when carnivores eat them, they turn into secondary producers because they are producing the energy for the meat - eaters since they ate the plants first. So this means that technically, secondary producers are also primary consumers.

5. What is the percentage of photosynthetically active radiation (PAR), in the incident solar radiation ?

(a) 100% **(b) 50%** **(c) 1–5%** **(d) 2–10%**

Sol. (b) Photosynthetically active radiation (PAR) is light of wavelength between 400 and 700 nm and is the portion of the light spectrum utilised by plants for photosynthesis. Of the incident solar radiation, less than 50 per cent of it is photosynthetically active radiation (PAR).

6. Distinguish between

(a) Grazing food chain and detritus food chain

(b) Production and decomposition

(c) Upright and inverted pyramid

(d) Food chain and food web

(e) Litter and detritus

(f) Primary and secondary productivity

Sol. (a) Grazing food chain and detritus food chain

S. No.	Grazing food chain	Detritus food chain
1.	This food chain begins with plants which are primary producers and ends with top carnivores which are tertiary or quaternary consumers.	This food chain begins with dead organic matter and then to organisms feeding on detritus called decomposers or saprophytes and ends with their predators.
2.	It depends on the sunlight for energy.	It depends on energy from dead organic remains.
3.	It fixes inorganic nutrients in the form of organic matter.	It returns inorganic nutrients to their reservoirs thus, important in recycling of nutrients.
4.	It supports detritus food chain by providing organic matter.	It supports grazing food chain by providing inorganic nutrients.

(b) Production and decomposition

S. No.	Production	Decomposition
1.	It is the process of synthesis of biomass or organic matter by producers.	It is the process of breakdown of complex organic matter into simple, inorganic substances by decomposers.
2.	Energy is trapped during production.	Energy is released during decomposition.
3.	It is anabolic process.	It is catabolic process.

(c) Upright and inverted pyramid

S. No.	Upright pyramid	Inverted pyramid
1.	This pyramid has broad base and with narrow apex.	This pyramid has narrow base and broad apex.
2.	Producers occupy the broad base and tertiary or quaternary consumers occupy the narrow apex.	Producers occupy the narrow apex and tertiary or quaternary consumers occupy the broad base.
3.	Example of such a pyramid is pyramid of energy, pyramid of biomass and pyramid of numbers.	Example of such a pyramid is pyramid of biomass in aquatic ecosystem and pyramid of numbers in tree-dominated ecosystem.
4.	Such pyramid is formed when number, biomass or energy of organisms decreases at successive trophic levels in a food chain.	Such pyramid is formed when number or biomass of organisms increases at successive trophic levels in a food chain.

(d) Food chain and food web

S. No.	Food chain	Food web
1.	Food chain consists of a linear series of organisms linked to each other based on their feeding relationship.	Food web consists of many interlinked food chains.
2.	It follows single pathway of flow of energy from producers to consumers.	It follows multiple pathways of flow of energy from producers to consumers.
3.	Organisms of higher trophic levels of a food chain feed upon one type of organism of lower trophic level.	Organisms of higher trophic levels in a food web have a number of organisms of lower trophic levels as alternate source of food.
4.	Change in population of an organism of any trophic level disrupts the food chain thus leading to instability of ecosystem.	Change in population of an organism of any trophic level does not disrupt the food web thus leading to stability of ecosystem.

(e) Litter and detritus

S. No.	Litter	Detritus
1.	Litter includes both biodegradable and non-biodegradable wastes generated above the ground.	Detritus includes biodegradable wastes generated both above and under the ground.
2.	Empty soft drink cans or bottles, potato chips bags, sweet wrappers, orange peels, etc. constitute litter.	Dead plant remains such as leaves, bark, flowers and dead remains of animals, including fecal matter constitute detritus.

(f) Primary and secondary productivity

S. No.	Primary productivity	Secondary productivity
1.	It is the rate of production of biomass or organic matter by producers.	It is the rate of formation of new organic matter by consumers.
2.	Fresh organic matter synthesis occurs from inorganic nutrients using radiant energy of sun.	Fresh organic matter synthesis occurs from pre-existing organic matter of producers or other consumers.

7. Describe the components of an ecosystem.

Sol. Ecosystems represent the interconnected nature of living organisms and their world. The *components of an ecosystem* can be divided into two categories : biotic and abiotic.

- *Biotic components* : These are the living components of an ecosystem that have a direct or indirect influence on other organisms in an environment. The life forms of an ecosystem help in the transfer and cycle of energy. They are grouped in terms of the means they use to get energy. Based on the source of their energy, biotic components can be further classified into the following:
  (i) Producers : They can synthesise their own food, e.g., green plants.
  (ii) Consumers : They do not synthesise their food. They depends on others for their food and may be classified into the following:
    - Primary consumer/herbivores : They feed on plants, e.g., insects, rats, squirrels, etc.
    - Secondary consumers or primary carnivores : Secondary consumers are those organisms that eat primary consumers for energy. Primary consumers are always herbivores, or organisms that only eat autotrophic plants. However, secondary consumers can either be carnivores or omnivores. E.g., frogs, birds, etc.

– Tertiary consumers or large carnivores : They feed on secondary consumers such as owl, fox, snakes, etc.

– Quaternary consumers : They are at the top of the food chain and eats tertiary consumers. They are also known as apex predators.

(iii) Decomposers : These organisms breakdown the dead bodies or waste products of plants and animals into simpler inorganic compounds. E.g., bacteria, fungi, earthworms.

- *Abiotic components* : These are the non-living or physical and chemical factors of an ecosystem. These are classified into following three categories:
  (i) Physical climatic factors : It includes light, temperature, wind, rain.
  (ii) Inorganic compounds : Like water, minerals and atmospheric gases, etc.
  (iii) Organic compounds : These includes organic substance present in the dead bodies of plant & animals.

8. Define ecological pyramids and describe with examples, pyramids of number and biomass.

Sol. *Ecological pyramid* is a graphical representation showing relationship among organisms of a food chain occupying different trophic levels expressed in terms of number, biomass or energy. In a pyramid, the base represents the producers or the first trophic level while the apex represents tertiary or top level consumer. Depending on the parameter used to represent an ecological pyramid, three types of pyramids are, pyramid of energy, pyramid of biomass and pyramid of number.

Pyramid of number : In this pyramid, the number of individuals of species of a food chain occupying different trophic levels is expressed. For example, the number of individuals in a food chain on grassland ecosystem is shown in the following pyramid of number:

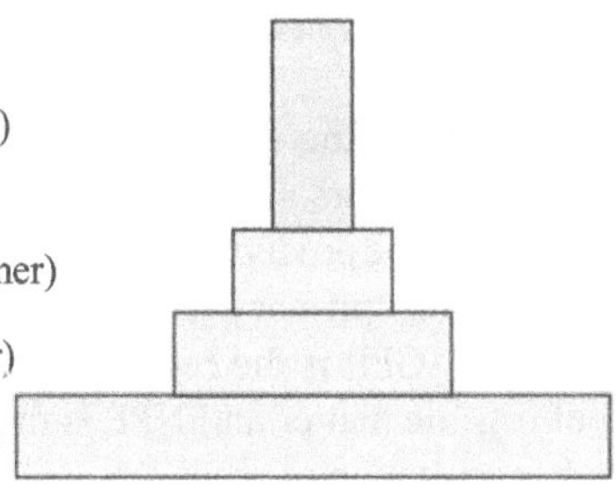

Trophic level	**Number of individuals**
TC (Tertiary consumer)	3
SC (Secondary consumer)	3,54,000
PC (Primary consumer)	708,000
PP (Primary producer)	5,842,000

From the pyramid, it is observed that as we move up the levels of the pyramid, the number of individuals in each level decreases. The producers form the largest number and hence are at the bottom of the pyramid. Such a pyramid of number is upright.

Inverted pyramid of number is obtained when the number of top carnivores is greater than the number of producers. For example, food chain in a forest ecosystem represented below results in an inverted pyramid of number.

Tree → Insects → Small birds → Large birds

Pyramid of biomass: In this pyramid, amount of biomass (total weight) present in a unit area of various trophic levels is expressed. For example, biomass of individuals of different trophic levels in a food chain on grassland ecosystem is shown in the following pyramid of biomass:

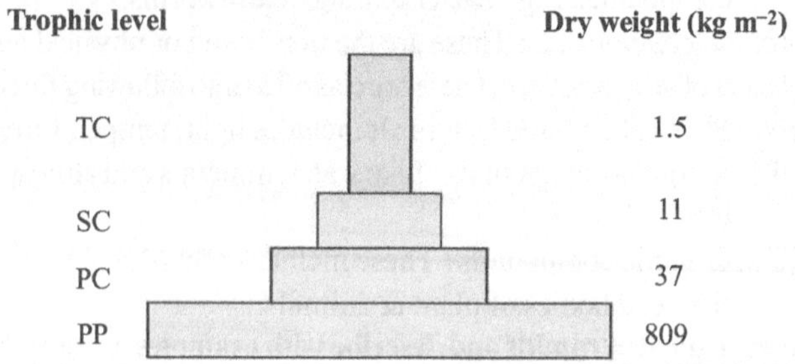

This pyramid indicates decrease of biomass in each tropical level from base to apex. The pyramid of biomass in sea is inverted because the biomass of fishes (primary consumer) far exceeds that of phytoplankton (primary producer).

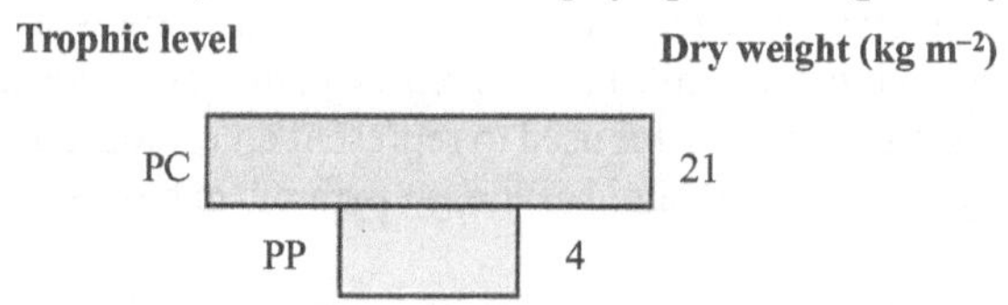

> **Note**
>
> *The concept of ecological pyramid was first introduced by Charles Elton, British Ecologist thus, ecological pyramids are also called Eltonian pyramids.*

9. What is primary productivity? Give brief description of factors that affect primary productivity.

Sol.
- *Primary productivity* is the rate of capture of solar energy or biomass production of the producers. It is expressed in terms of gm-2 yr-1 or (kcal m-2) yr-1 to compare the productivity of different ecosystems. It is divided into two types: gross primary productivity (GPP) and net primary productivity (NPP). GPP is the rate of capture of solar energy or total production of organic matter and NPP is the remaining biomass or the energy left after utilisation of producers.
- *Factors affecting primary productivity are*:
  (i) Availability of nutrients which varies in different types of ecosystem.
  (ii) Photosynthetic capacity of plants.
  (iii) The plant species inhabiting a particular area.
  (iv) Environmental factor.

10. Define decomposition and describe the processes and products of decomposition.

Sol. • *Decomposition* is the process of breakdown of dead or waste complex organic matter into inorganic substances such as carbon dioxide, water and nutrients by decomposers. Decomposition is both physical and chemical in nature.

- *Processes involved in decomposition* are as follows:
  (i) *Fragmentation*: It is the first process during which detritivores such as earthworm break down detritus into smaller particles. Due to this process, the surface area of detritus is greatly increased.
  (ii) *Leaching*: During this process, water-soluble inorganic nutrients present in fragmented detritus go down into the soil horizon along with percolating water and get precipitated as unavailable salts.
  (iii) *Catabolism*: In this process, bacteria and fungi secrete extracellular enzymes that degrade detritus into simpler inorganic substances.
  (iv) *Humification*: It is the process of accumulation of a dark coloured amorphous substance called humus which serves as a reservoir of nutrients. It is highly resistant to microbial action and undergoes decomposition at an extremely slow rate.
  (v) *Mineralisation*: During this process, inorganic nutrients are released in the soil by further degradation of humus by some microbes.
- *Products of decomposition* are water, carbon dioxide and nutrients such as nitrogen, phosphorous, calcium, potassium, sulphur, etc.

11. Give an account of energy flow in an ecosystem.

Sol. *Energy flow* refers to the flow of energy in an ecosystem through a series of organisms of a food chain or web. It flows through different organisms in the following manner:

- Sun is the only source of energy for all ecosystems on Earth. Solar energy enters the ecosystem through the process of photosynthesis. Plants and photosynthetic bacteria (autotrophs) called primary producers capture Sun's radiant energy to make food from simple inorganic materials. All animals depend on plants for their food needs directly or indirectly.
- No energy that is trapped into an organism remains in it forever. The energy trapped by the producer, hence, is either passed on to a consumer through the beginning of grazing food chain or on to decomposers in case of death of the plant thus, beginning a detritus food chain or web.
- The energy stored in plants is passed on to the primary consumers (herbivores) in the food chain when they consume the plants as food. When these herbivores are consumed by carnivores of the first order (secondary consumers), energy is transfer occurs from herbivores to carnivores. Finally, when tertiary consumers consume the carnivores, again energy will be transferred. Thus, there is unidirectional flow of energy from the sun to producers and then to consumers.

- Based on the source of their nutrition or food, organisms occupy a specific place in the food chain called trophic level. Producers belong to the first trophic level, herbivores (primary consumer) to the second and carnivores (secondary consumer) to the third.
- The transfer of energy follows 10 per cent law according to which only 10 per cent of the energy is transferred to each trophic level from the lower trophic level *i.e.*, the amount of energy decreases at successive trophic levels due to loss of energy in the form of heat.

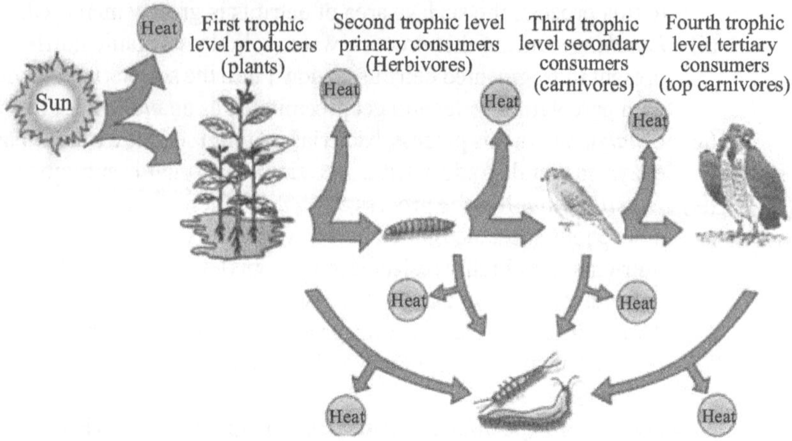

Fig. : Energy flow through different trophic levels

> **Note**
>
> *The Ten percent law for the transfer of energy from one trophic level to the next was introduced by Lindemann (1942). According to this law, during the transfer of energy from organic food from one trophic level to the next, only about ten percent of energy from organic matter is stored as flesh. The remaining is lost during transfer, broken down in respiration, or lost to incomplete digestion by higher trophic levels.*

12. Write important features of a sedimentary cycle in an ecosystem.

Sol. Sedimentary cycle is the movement of non-gaseous nutrient elements such as phosphorous, calcium and sulphur through the various components of an ecosystem.

The *important features of such cycles* are as follows:

(i) They have Earth's crust as their reservoir.

(ii) These cycles consist of two phases, solution and rock phases. In the solution phase, minerals are released from Earth's crust in the form of salts due to weathering and some of these salts dissolve in water, pass through a series of organisms, and ultimately reach the deep seas, where they move out of circulation indefinitely. In the rock phase, other salts deposit out as sediment and rock in shallow seas, eventually to be weathered and recycled.

(iii) These cycles are slower than gaseous cycles.

(iv) Such cycles are less perfect system because elements get trapped in the reservoir pool and go out of circulation for long periods.

13. Outline salient features of carbon cycling in an ecosystem.

Sol. Carbon cycle is a gaseous biogeochemical cycle with its reservoir in ocean, atmosphere and fossil fuels.

Salient features of carbon cycle are:

(i) It occurs through atmosphere, ocean and through living and dead organisms.

(ii) Producers use CO_2 through photosynthesis in the presence of sunlight to form their food in the form of carbohydrate which is transferred to other organisms through food chains. Thus, it is fixed in the biosphere.

(iii) It returns to the atmosphere as CO_2 through respiratory activities of the producers and consumers and processing of waste materials and dead organic matter of land or oceans by decomposers.

(iv) Some amount of the fixed carbon is lost to sediments and removed from circulation.

(v) Burning of wood, forest fire and combustion of organic matter, fossil fuel and volcanic activity also release CO_2 in the atmosphere.

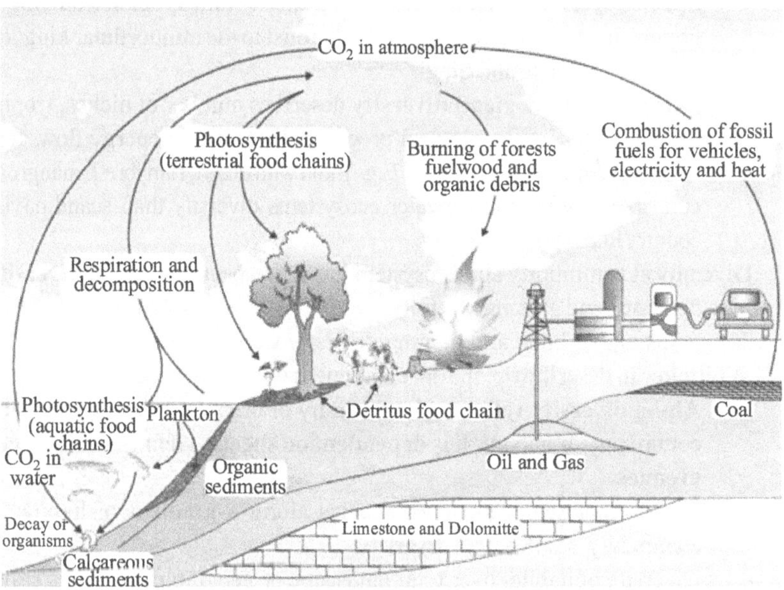

Fig. : Carbon cycle

Chapter 15 BIODIVERSITY AND CONSERVATION

CHAPTER AT A GLANCE

- **Biodiversity or biological diversity** is the occurrence of different types of ecosystem, different species of organisms with their biotypes & genes adapted to different climates, environments along with their interactions & processes.
- Biodiversity includes three inter-related hierarchial levels. These are **genetic diversity, species diversity & community/ecosystem/ecological diversity**.
  - **Genetic diversity** refers to variation of genes within species both among geographically separated populations and among individual of single population. These differences can be in between alleles, in entire genes or in chromosomal structures.
  - **Species diversity** refer to variety of species within a region from micro-organisms such as virus, bacteria and protist to the multicellular kingdom of plants, animals and fungi.
  - **Ecosystem (ecological) diversity** describes number of niches, trophic levels and various ecological processes that sustain energy flow, food web and recycling of nutrients, E.g., India with desert, rain forest, mangrove, coral reef, wetland has greater ecosystems diversity than scandinavian country like Norway.
- Diversity at community and ecosystem has 3 perspectives: **alpha diversity**, **beta diversity**, and **gamma diversity**.
- The terms alpha, beta, and gamma diversity were all introduced by **R. H. Whittaker to describe the spatial component of biodiversity**.
  - **Alpha diversity** refers to the diversity of organism sharing the same community or habitat. It is **dependent on species richness and species evenness.**
  - The rate of replacement of species along a gradient of habitat or community is called **beta diversity**.
  - Diversity of habitat over total landscape or geographical area is called **gamma diversity**.
- Biodiversity varies with change in latitude or altitude. Biodiversity increases, as we move from high to low latitude as (*i.e.,* from poles to equator).
- The relation between species richness and area having wide variety of taxa is **rectangular hyperbola**.

- The number of species per unit area is called **species richness** and the number of individuals of different species represents **species evenness**.
- If individuals of a species remain alive only in captivity or other human controlled conditions, the species is said to be **extinct in wild**.
- A species is said to be **locally extinct** if it is no longer found in area, once it inhabited, but is still found somewhere else in wild.
- A species is said to be **ecologically extinct** if it persists at such reduced numbers that its effect on other species in community are negligible. For instance, few tigers remain in wild that their impact on prey population is insignificant.
- **Loss of biodiversity or biodiversity loss** is the extinction of species (plant or animal) worldwide, and also the local reduction or loss of species in a certain habitat.
- The International Union for Conservation of Nature **(IUCN)** was established in the year 1964 to **maintain Red Data Book**.
- **Red data book** is a source document which maintains the record of all the rare and endangered species of animals, plants and fungi as well as some local subspecies that exist within the territory of the state or country.
- IUCN (Red list, 2004) documents the extinctions of 784 species in which 338 are vertebrates, 359 are invertebrates and 87 plants in the last 500 years.
- **Major causes of loss of biodiversity** are - habitat destruction, habitat fragmentation, habitat degradation & pollution, introduction of exotic species, over exploitation and co-extinction.
- **Introduction of exotic species**, increased levels of diseases, and excessive exploitation of particular species causes significant biodiversity losses.
- Disease causing micro-organisms, if introduced to new virgin areas may cause epidemics and native species are eliminated completely.
- **Over exploitation** includes the activities like over hunting, over fishing, illegal trade of wildlife and excessive logging. It threatens 1/3rd of endangered vertebrates in the world, as well as other species. Such as whales, steller's sea cow and passenger pigeon. Even if a species is not completely eliminated by over exploitation, the population size may become too small that the species is unable to recover.
- Presently, **12%** of all bird species, **23%** of all mammal species, **32%** of all amphibian species and **31%** of all gymnosperm species in the world face the threat of extinction.
- The current species extinction rates are estimated to be 100-1,000 times faster than in pre-human times.
- **Threatened Species** = Endangered + Vulnerable + Rare
- Species with small world population that are not presently endangered or vulnerable but are at risk, are called **rare species**. E.g., Venus fly trap only in Savannah of coastal plains of Carolina in East U.S.A.

BIODIVERSITY CONSERVATION

- **Biodiversity conservation** is basically aimed at protection, enhancement and scientific management of the biodiversity.
- It is important to conserve biodiversity because of its several benefits it offers that are essential to live. It provides biological resources, ecosystem services, social and spiritual benefits.
- IUCN and WWF are leading International Organisations concerned with biodiversity conservation.
- **"The earth Summit"** held in Rio de Jeneiro in 1992 called upon all nations to take appropriate measures for conservation of biodiversity and sustainable utilisation of its benefits.
- There are **2 basic methods of biodiversity conservation: *In situ* (on site) and *Ex situ* (off site).**

In situ conservation

- *In situ* method provides protection to total ecosystem. It includes protection of a group of typical ecosystems through a network of protected areas.
- Example of protected areas are **national park, wild life sancturies** and **biosphere reserve.**
- The **first national park in India is Hailey national park**. It was set up in 1935 in the foot hills of Himalayas in Uttar Pradesh.
- **Hot spots** are the richest and most threatened reservoir of plants and animals life on earth.
- The **concept of hot spot of biodiversity** was developed by **Norman Myers** (in 1988) to designate priority area for in situ conservation.
- 25 terrestrial hot spots for conservation of biodiversity have been identified world wide.

  Among 25 hot spots of world, 2 are located in India, which are Western Ghat and Eastern Himalayas. These are regions of accelerated habitat loss.
- Biodiversity hotspots region have very high levels of species richness and high degree of endemism (species are confined to that region and are not found anywhere else).

Ex - situ conservation

- It a set of conservation techniques which involves the transfer of a target species away from its native habitat.
- **Concept of ex situ conservation** was developed earlier before its official adoption under the Convention on Biological Diversity signed in 1992 in **Rio de Janeiro**.
- It includes **botanical gardens, zoos, conservation stands** and **gene, pollen seed, seedling, tissue culture and DNA banks.**
- India has 10 biogeographical regions, 89 national parks, 500 wild life sanctuaries, 14 biosphere reserves, 6 wetlands and 35 world heritage sites.

EXERCISE

1. Name the three important components of biodiversity.

Sol. Biodiversity refers to heterogeneity existing at all levels of biological organisation ranging from macromolecules within cells to biomes.

Three components of biodiversity are:

(i) Genetic diversity – It refers to total genetic information contained in the individuals of plants, animals and microorganisms.

(ii) Species diversity – It comprises of the number of different species that are present in a region.

(iii) Ecological diversity – It refers to variety of habitats, biotic communities and ecological processes in an area.

2. How do ecologists estimate the total number of species present in the world?

Sol. The ecologists estimate the total number of species present in the world using the statistical methods because the number of species is too large. They make a significant comparison of species richness of exhaustively studied groups of insects of the temperate and tropical regions and extrapolate this ratio to other groups of animals and plants to calculate gross estimate of the total number of species existing on the earth.

3. Give three hypotheses for explaining why tropics show greatest levels of species richness.

Sol. Tropics harbour more species than temperate or polar areas. The *three hypotheses explaining the reason for greatest species richness in tropics* are as follows:

(i) *Constant environment* : Tropical environments, unlike temperate ones, are less seasonal, relatively more constant and predictable. Such constant environments promote niche specialisation and lead to a greater species diversity.

(ii) *Prolonged evolutionary time* : Temperate regions are subjected to frequent glaciations in the past and resulted in extinction of the species. In contrast, tropical regions have remained relatively undisturbed for millions of years and thus, had a long evolutionary time for species diversification.

(iii) *Higher productivity* : Tropics receive more solar energy which contributes to higher productivity which, in turn, contributes indirectly to greater diversity.

4. What is the significance of the slope of regression in a species – area relationship?

Sol. The species-area relationship describes the relationship between the part of a habitat and the number of species found within that area. On a logarithmic scale, the relationship between species richness and area for a wide variety of taxa (angiosperm plants, birds, bats, freshwater fishes) is a straight line described by the following equation:

$$\log S = \log C + Z \log A$$

where,

S = Species richness

A = Area

Z = slope of the line (regression coefficient)

C = Y-intercept

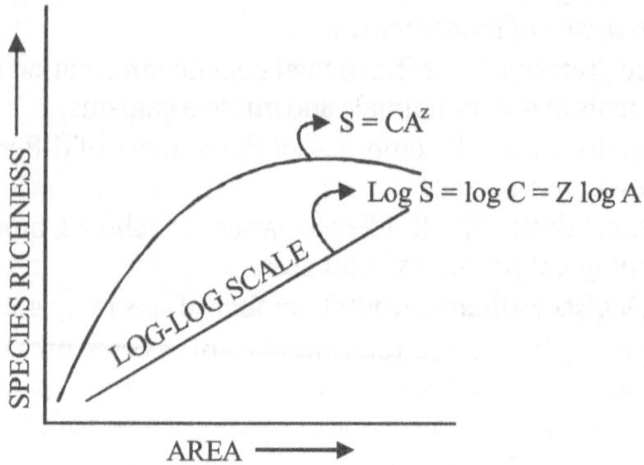

Fig.: Species - area relationship

In this equation, the slope of a regression line (Z) represents the rate of change in species richness as area changes. It is very important for determining species-area relationship. On analysing species-area relationship, regardless of the taxonomic group or the region, the value of Z lies in the range of 0.1 to 0.2 for smaller area whereas Z ranges from 0.6 to 1.2 for large areas. It *signifies that species richness increases with increasing area of observation.*

In larger areas, the slope of regression coefficient becomes steeper.

> **Note**
>
> *Steeper slopes signifies that number of species found increases faster than the area explored in very large areas like the entire continents.*

5. What are the major causes of species losses in a geographical region?

Sol. Loss of biodiversity means extinction of species. Species are lost in a geographical region due to the following reasons:

(i) *Habitat loss and fragmentation* : Habitats of various organisms are altered or destroyed by uncontrolled and unsustainable human activities (such as deforestation, slash and burn agriculture, mining, and urbanisation). This will lead to breaking up of the habitat into small pieces, which effect the movement of migratory animals and also, decrease the genetic exchange between populations leading to a declination of species.

(ii) *Over-exploitation* : Overexploitation can lead to the destruction of the resource. Due to over-hunting and over-exploitation of various plants and animals many species have become endangered or extinct. For example: Tiger and Steller's sea cow, the passenger pigeon).

(iii) *Alien species invasions* : Accidental or intentional introduction of non-native species into a habitat has led to the declination or extinction of indigenous species. For example, the Nile perch introduced in Lake Victoria in Kenya led to the extinction of more than two hundred species of native fish in the lake.

(iv) *Co-extinction* : In a native habitat, one species is connected to the other in an intricate network. The extinction of one species causes the extinction of other species, which is associated with it in an obligatory way. Co-extinction is especially common when a keystone species goes extinct. For example, the extinction of the host will cause the extinction of its parasites.

6. How is biodiversity important for ecosystem functioning?

Sol. *Biodiversity is important for ecosystem functioning* because,

(i) It contributes to productivity. High biodiversity makes the ecosystem more stable in productivity and more resistant towards disturbances such as alien species invasions and floods.

(ii) It cause more efficient recycling of energy and matter.

(iii) It has many alternative pathways for survival under diverse conditions.

(iv) If an ecosystem is rich in biodiversity, then the ecological balance should be maintained and would not get affected. Rich biodiversity provides alternatives available at each trophic level. All organisms are linked in food chains and interact with their abiotic environment in such a way so as to keep the natural cycles going and make the ecosystems self – sustaining units. Therefore, it can be concluded that if an ecosystem is rich in species, then there will be other food alternatives at each trophic level which would not allow any organism to die due to the absence of their food resource.

7. What are sacred groves? What is their role in conservation?

Sol.
- *Sacred groves* are areas of forest or trees which are regenerated around places of worship. These areas are dedicated to local deities or ancestral spirits and are protected by local communities through social traditions and taboos that incorporate spiritual and ecological values. These groves are found in Rajasthan, Western Ghats of Karnataka, and Maharashtra, Meghalaya, and Madhya Pradesh. Deforestation is strictly prohibited in this region by tribals.
- *Role in conservation* : Sacred groves give much ecological and genetically significance and help in the protection of many rare, threatened, and endemic species of plants and animals found in that area. It also provides vital ecosystem services to local people.

8. Among the ecosystem services are control of floods and soil erosion. How is this achieved by the biotic components of the ecosystem?

Sol. Ecosystem services are products or benefits given by ecosystem processes to the environment for its purification, beauty, biodiversity, protection of natural resources, habitat to wild life and tribals, protection of soils, CO_2 - O_2 balance, retention of water against floods, drought and pollution.

The biotic components of an ecosystem include the living organisms such as plants, animals, fungi and microorganisms that make up ecological communities. Plants play a vital role in the control of floods and soil erosion. Their roots bind the soil particles firmly and in this way they do not allow the top soil to be drifted away by winds or moving water. Roots of plants also make the soil porous and allow water to go into the soil. They also increase the soil fertility and biodiversity.

9. The species diversity of plants (22 per cent) is much less than that of animals (72 per cent). What could be the explanations to how animals achieved greater diversification?

Sol. Species diversity refers to the variety of species within a region which is less in plants as compared to animals.

- More than 70 percent of species recorded on the Earth are animals and only 22 percent species are plants. There is quiet a large difference in their percentage. This is because animals have adapted themselves to ensure their survival in changing environments in comparison to plants.
- *Animals achieved such greater diversification due to the following reasons* :
  (i) Most animals possess simple or complex nervous system to control and coordinate various activities. They possess receptors to receive against them. Most of their responses are adaptive and ensure their survival in changing environmental conditions. They, therefore, have evolved to reveal much higher species diversity than plants who do not possess nervous system and respond differently against environment stimuli.
  (ii) Similarly, repeated body segments with paired appendages and external cuticles have made insects versatile and given them the ability to survive in various environments as compared to other life forms.

10. Can you think of a situation where we deliberately want to make a species extinct? How would you justify it?

Sol.
- Yes, there are different types of parasites and disease-causing microbes that we deliberately want to eradicate from the Earth. Since these micro-organisms are harmful to human beings, scientists are working hard to fight against them.
- Scientists have been able to eliminate small pox virus from the world with the help of vaccinations. This shows that humans want to make these species extinct and make this world disease free. Several other eradication programmes such as polio and Hepatitis B vaccinations are aimed to eliminate these disease-causing microbes. Since, such micro-organisms are harmful to the human society, these attempt is justified.
- Further, such micro-organisms are not essential components (producers or decomposers) of any ecosystem and losing one or few such organisms would not affect the functioning of ecosystem.

16 ENVIRONMENTAL ISSUES

Chapter

CHAPTER AT A GLANCE

- **Pollution** is any undesirable change in physical, chemical or biological character of air, land, water or soil.
- **Pollutants** are the elements, molecules and particles involved in pollution.
- The major kinds of pollution, usually classified by environment, are air pollution, water pollution, and land pollution.

AIR POLLUTION

- Air pollution refers to the undesirable change occurring in air causing harmful effects on man and domesticated species.
- The chemical compounds that lower the air quality are usually referred to as **air pollutants**. These compounds may be found in the air in two major forms: in a gaseous form (as gases), and in a solid form (as particulate matter suspended in the air).
- **Primary air pollutant** are those poisonous gases and undesirable substance which are released by burning fossil fuels.
- The **primary air pollutants** are soot released from unburned fuel, sulphur dioxide (SO_2), benzopyrene (hydrocarbon) released from cigarette smoke, ammonia (NH_3), oxides of nitrogen., carbon monoxide (CO), lead (Pb).
- **Secondary air pollutants** are poisonous substance formed from primary air pollutants. In bright sun light nitrogen, nitrogen oxides, hydrocarbons and O_2 interact to produce more powerful photochemical oxidants like ozone (O_3), peroxyacetyl nitrate (PAN), aldehydes, sulphuric acid, peroxides, etc. All these constitute photochemical smog, which retard photosynthesis in plants.
- **Causes of air pollution** are
  - Industrialisation and automobile exhaustion.
  - Overpopulation, deforestation, nuclear explosion and explosives used in war and fireworks.
  - Volcanic eruption, electric storm and solarflares, forest fire, dust storms.
  - Pollen, spores, cyst, bacteria and marshy flares gases (methane, CH_4).
- **Effect of CO:** CO (carbon monoxide) is the most poisonous gas and is released from motor vehicles & industries. CO combines with haemoglobin and reduces oxygen carrying capacity of haemoglobin.
- **CO_2** (carbon dioxide) causes **greenhouse effects**.

- **Effects of NO and NO_2**
  - Nitrogen monoxide (NO), like CO, lowers oxygen carrying capacity of blood.
  - Nitrogen dioxide (NO_2), on contact with H_2O vapour in air, forms a highly corrosive nitric acid (HNO_3), which irritates eyes, nose, lungs.
  - Causes defoliation and necrosis.
- **Effects of SO_2 and SO_3**
  - They causes respiratory diseases like asthma, bronchitis and emphysema.
  - SO_2 causes chlorosis, necrosis of vegetation, metabolic inhibition of growth reduction.
  - SO_2 and SO_3 makes sulphurous acid (H_2SO_3) and sulphuric acid (H_2SO_4) respectively. It may precipitate as rain or snow, producing **acid rain**.
- **Hydrocarbons or volatile organic carbon** are produced due to incomplete combustion of fuel in automobiles. They are also formed by bacterial decomposition of organic matter.
- Methane, the most aboundant hydrocarbon in atmosphere is evolved from soil in flooded rice fields & swamps.
- Benzene and its derivative such as formaldehyde are carcinogenic.
- **Particulate pollutants** are added to air by industries and automobiles, operations like blasting, drilling, crushing, grinding and mixing. They can also be added by living organisms like pollen, spores, cysts and bacteria.
- **Control of air pollution**
  - Good quality fuel like lead free or low sulphur should be used in motor vehicles.
  - Installation of equipments like gravity settling tanks or porous filters and **electrostatic precipitator** can minimise air pollution. The precipitator removes smaller particles.
  - Vehicles based on compressed natural gas (CNG) should be introduced. Delhi become the first city of the world to use CNG for public transport system.
- **In 1987, the Air (Prevention and Control of Pollution) Act** was amended to include noise as a source of air pollution. In India this act came into force in 1981.

WATER POLLUTION

- Water pollution is the deterioration of the quality of water due to addition of foreign substances, factors (heat) & deprivation that makes it health hazard, unfit for human use & aquatic organisms.
- **Sources of water pollution**
  - Industrial discharge of chemical wastes & byproducts.
  - Discharge of poorly treated or untreated sewage.
  - Surface run off containing pesticides.
  - Slash & burn farming practice, which is often an element within shifting cultivation agricultural system.

- **Oil pollution:** Oil is a source of pollution in sea-water. Oil pollution is due to ship accidents, loading and discharging of oil at the harbour, oil refineries and off-shore oil production. Degree of impurity of after due to organic matter is measured in terms of BOD (Biochemical Oxygen Demand). Oil cannot dissolve in water and forms a thick sludge in water. This suffocates fish, gets caught in the feathers of marine birds stopping them from flying and blocks light from photosynthetic aquatic plants.

- **BOD** refers to amount of dissolved oxygen needed by bacteria in decomposing the organic waste of water. It is expressed as milligram of O_2/ litre of waste in water. A pure water should have BOD < 1500 mg/litre.
- When large amount of sewage is dumped into water, the BOD will increase.
- **Chemical oxygen demand (COD)** test is aimed to determine the amount of oxygen needed to oxidise all pollution materials.
- The value of COD is much higher than BOD.
- Phosphorus and nitrates dissolved in H_2O act as nutrients and accelerate the growth of algae (**algal bloom**) that forms a mat on water surface. This increased productivity is called **eutrophication.**
- The phenonmenon through which certains pollutants gets accumulated in tissues in increasing concentration along the food chain is called **biological magnification**.
- Polluted water is treated in effluent treatment plant before their release in the water bodies. Three **main steps in sewage treatment are-**
  - **Primary treatment:** It involves physical treatments such as sedimentation, floatation, fragmentation and filteration.
  - **Secondary treatment:** There are two ways - anoxic (through the action of anoxic micro-organisms and macromolecules) and aerobic (it occurs by two ways - trickling filter method and activated sludge methods).
  - **Tertiary treatment:** It includes removal of nitrates and phosphates.

SOLID WASTE

- Solid wastes, any discarded or abandoned materials, can be solid, liquid, semi-solid or containerized gaseous material.
- Types of solid waste are: municipal solid waste, industrial solid waste and biomedical waste or hospital waste.
- **Modern landfill site** is a disposal site for solid waste where the waste is buried between layers of soil, filling in low lying ground.
- **Electronic waste or e-waste**, is a term for electronic products that have become unwanted, non-working or obsolete, and have essentially reached the end of their useful life.
- E-waste can be treated or destroyed by **incineration** (burning in presence of oxygen), and **landfills** (in which the e-wastes are dumped in a trench or depression after compaction and covered with dirt every day). But this method can be dangerous as it can leach lead and other substances in soil and groundwater and contaminate them.
- **Polyblends** is a fine powder of recycled modified plastics. It has been used in the development of roads in Bangalore.

AGRO-CHEMICALS AND THEIR EFFECTS AND RADIOACTIVE WASTE

- Agrochemicals are chemical used in agriculture. It includes chemical fertilisers, herbicides, and insecticides.
- **Radioactive waste** is a type of waste in gas, liquid or solid form that contains radioactive nuclear substance.
- **Organic farming** is a form of agriculture, which avoids or largely excludes the use of synthetic fertilisers and pesticides, plant growth regulators & livestock feed additives.
- Organic farmers rely on crop rotation, crop residues, animal manures & mechanical cultivation to maintain soil productivity, to supply plant nutrients & to control weeds etc.

GREENHOUSE EFFECT AND OZONE HOLE

- Greenhouse gases such as CO_2, CH_4, N_2O and CFC's present in atmosphere radiate part of radio wave radiations emitted by earth back to the earth. This downflux is called **greenhouse flux** which keeps the earth warm and the phenomenon is called **greenhouse effect**.
- Due to increased/enhanced green house effect there is increase in global mean temperature known as **global warming**. The global warming has many fold effects as – effect on climate, sea level change, effects on range of species distribution; food production.
- **Control of greenhouse effect**
  - Less use of fossil fuel.
  - Improving efficiency of energy usage.
  - Reducing deforestation.
  - Increasing the vegetation cover, mainly the forests for photosynthesis.
  - Decreasing down growth of human population.
  - Developing substitutes for CFC.
- **Ozone layer** (discovered by Charles fabry and Henri Buisson, french physicists in 1913) in stratosphere acts as **ozone shield** and protects earth biota from harmful effect of UV radiation.
- **Ozone (O_3) depletion** refers to the phenomenon of reduction in the amount of ozone in the stratosphere.
- Ozone hole is **usually present from September to November** each year.
- CFC, nitrogen oxides & hydrocarbons are responsible for O_3 depletion. Ozone layer depletion has various negative effects on atmosphere. UV radiation increases more on earth. In human it causes skin cancer cataract, reducing the functioning of immune systems.

DEFORESTATION AND DEGRADATION OF NATURAL RESOURCES

- **Soil erosion** may be defined as depletion of fertile top soil by over-cultivation, unrestricted grazing, deforestation and poor irrigation practices, resulting in arid patches of land. When large barren patches extend and meet over, the desert is created. Without soil and plants, the land becomes desert like and unable to support life. This process is called **desertification**. It is major problem now a days particularly due to increased urbanization.

- **Waterlogging and soil salinity** retards growth of crop damaging agriculture. Irrigation without proper drainage of water leads to waterlogging in soil. Beside affecting crops, waterlogging draws salt to surface of soil. The salt is then deposited as thin crust on land surface or start collecting at roots of the plants.
- **Deforestation** is the conversion of forested area to non-forested one.
- **Consequence of deforestation** is greenhouse effect, loss of biodiversity due to habitat destruction, disturbance in hydrological cycles, soil erosion and desertification in extreme cases.
- **Conservation of forests** aim at management of forests in such a way so as to maintain them at optimum form and derive optimum sustainable benefit for present as well as future generations.
- **Joint Forest Management Concept** was adopted considering the extraordinary courage and dedication the local people showed in protecting the wildlife through the movements like Bishnoi's is movement in Jodhpur and Chipko Movement in Garhwal Himalayas.

EXERCISE

1. What are the various constituents of domestic sewage? Discuss the effects of sewage discharge on a river.

Sol. Domestic sewage is composed of human body waste and sullage which is the waste water resulting from kitchen, bathroom and laundry sources.

- *Constitute of domestic sewage*

  Domestic sewage contains four kinds of impurities:

  (i) *Suspended solids* : They are soil particles such as sand and silt.

  (ii) *Colloidal particles* : They are inorganic and organic materials such as faecal matter, bacteria, paper and cloth.

  (iii) *Dissolved solids* : They are nitrates, phosphates, ammonia, sodium, calcium and other nutrients.

  (iv) *Pathogens (disease causing microbes)* : Domestic sewage has pathogens of various diseases such as typhoid, cholera, dysentery, diarrhoea, etc.

- *Effects of sewage discharge on a river* : Sewage may affect the aquatic environment by increasing the level of biological oxygen demand (BOD) and formation of algal bloom. Effect of sewage discharge on river are as follow :

  (i) Eutrophication.

  (ii) Growth of pathogenic bacteria.

  (iii) Ageing of river where slit and decaying matters start accumulating and filling river.

(iv) *Increase in BOD.* When organic wastes from the sewage enter the water bodies, they become the food source for micro-organisms (such as algae and bacteria) and thereby increase their population. Here, they utilise most of the dissolved oxygen for their metabolism. This results in an increase in the levels of biological oxygen demand (BOD) in river water and results in the death of aquatic organisms.

(v) Destruction of flora and fauna of that river.

(vi) The nutrients in the water lead to the growth of planktonic algal, causing *algal bloom*. This causes deterioration of water quality and fish mortality.

2. List all the wastes that you generate, at home, school or during your trips to other places. Could you very easily reduce the generation of these wastes? Which would be difficult or rather impossible to reduce?

Sol. • Wastes generated at

- *home* include plastic bags, paper napkin, toiletries, kitchen wastes (such as peelings of vegetables and fruits, tea leaves), domestic sewage, glass, etc.
- *schools* include waste paper, plastics, vegetable and fruit peels, food wrappings, sewage etc.
- *trips or picnics* include plastic, paper, vegetable and fruit peels, disposable cups, plates, spoons etc.

• *Yes, we can easily reduce these generated waste* through judicious use of material by changing our habits & life styles. It can also be reduced if we carefully use or recycle the above-mentioned waste materials generated at home, school or trips.

• *Waste materials which can be easily reduced and recycled* are paper, plastic and glass. Wastage of paper can be minimised by writing on its both sides also. Also, substituting plastics bags with biodegradable jute bags can reduce wastes generated at home, school, or during trips. Domestic sewage can be reduced by optimising the use of water while bathing, cooking, and other household activities.

• *Waste material which is difficult to reduce* are non biodegradable waste. Non- biodegradable wastes such as plastic, metal, broken glass, etc. are difficult to decompose because micro-organisms do not have the ability to decompose them.

3. Discuss the causes and effects of global warming. What measures need to be taken to control global warming?

Sol. • Global warming is defined as a gradual rise in the average temperature of the Earth's surface. Increase in atmospheric concentration of green house gases has resulted in rise of atmospheric temperature by 0.6°C (global warming) in the 20th century. This has been confirmed by intergovernmental panel on climatic change (IPCC) in its reports of 1991 and 1992. This predictable change in near future may affect climate, sea level, range of species distribution, food production as well as fisheries resources in the oceans.

- *Causes of global warming*
  (i) Increase in concentration of greenhouse gases.
  (ii) Increase of automobile and use of fossil fuel.
  (iii) Deforestation and change in land use.
  (iv) CFC and aerosol emission from refrigerator and aeroplane.
  (v) Increased particulate matter in lower atmosphere.
- *Effects of global warming*
  (i) CO_2 fertilisation effect.
  (ii) Many species of plants, being sensitive to temperature will die with sudden rise in temperature and their place will be taken over by scrub vegetation.
  (iii) Loss of biodiversity.
  (iv) Rise in sea level and change of precepitation and local climate conditions.
  (v) Possibilities of drought and floods.
  (vi) Erruption of plant disease and pests.
  (vii) Change in rainfall pattern.
- *Methods that can reduce the atmospheric concentration of greenhouses gases* are as follows:
  (i) Reducing the greenhouse gas emission by limiting the use of fossil fuels, and by developing alternative renewable sources of energy (wind energy, solar energy etc.)
  (ii) Increasing the vegetation cover, mainly the forests, for photosynthetic utilisation of CO_2.
  (iii) Minimising the use of nitrogen fertilisers in agriculture for reducing N_2O emissions.
  (iv) Developing substitutes for chlorofluorocarbons.

4. Match the items given in column A and B.

	Column A		Column B
(a)	Catalytic converter	(i)	Particulate matter
(b)	Electrostatic precipitator	(ii)	Carbon monoxide and nitrogen oxides
(c)	Earmuffs	(iii)	High noise level
(d)	Landfills	(iv)	Solid wastes

Sol. (a) – (ii) *Catalytic converter* is a device on a car that reduces the amount of poisonous gas (as carbon monoxide, unburned hydrocarbons, and oxides of nitrogen) that is released from the exhaust. It converts harmful pollutants into less harmful emissions by catalysing a redox reaction (an oxidation and a reduction reaction) before they ever leave the car's exhaust system.

(b) – (i) *Electrostatic converter* is a filtration device. It removes suspended dust particles from a gas or exhaust by applying a high-voltage electrostatic charge and collecting the particles on charged plates. It can remove over 99 per cent particulate matter present in the exhaust from a thermal power plant.

(c) – (iii) *Earmuffs* are a pair of ear covering which protects it from loud noise. They consist of a thermoplastic or metal head-band that fits over the top or back of the head, and a cushion or cup at each end, to cover the external ears.

(d) – (iv) *Landfills* may be defined as an area which built up from deposits of solid refuse in layers covered by soil.

5. Write critical notes on the following:

(a) Eutrophication (b) Biological magnification

(c) Groundwater depletion and ways for its replenishment

Sol. (a) Eutrophication

- It is an natural process in lakes, occurring as they age through geological time.
- Eutrophication is the process by which a body of water becomes enriched in dissolved nutrients (such as nitrogen and phosphates) that stimulate the growth of aquatic plant life usually resulting in the depletion of dissolved oxygen leading to the death of animal life.
- As a result, it causes a tremendous increase in the primary productivity of the ecosystem. This leads to an increased growth of algae, resulting into algal blooms (caused by the phosphates in detergents, fertilisers, and sewage). Later, the decomposition of these algae depletes the supply of oxygen, leading to the death of another aquatic animal life.

(b) Biological magnification

- Biomagnifications is defined as the increase in concentration of pollutants or harmful substances that occur in the food chain due to the following consequencs:
  (i) Persistence (means it can't be broken down by environmental process).
  (ii) Bioenergetic in the food chain.
  (iii) Low rate of internal degradation or excretion of the substances.

  The maximum concentration is accumulated at the top carnivore's level of food chain.
- Biological magnification depends on two factors: chemicals that are soluble in fat, but insoluble in water; and, chemicals that either are not broken down or are broken down slowly in the environment.
- This phenomenon can be seen in the case of mercury or DDT. The concentration of mercury/DDT increases at the successive trophic levels.
- To illustrate the process of biological magnification, the example of the pesticide DDT moving through an aquatic food chain can be given. DDT is insoluble in water, soluble in fat and breaks down slowly in the environment.

  High concentration of DDT (dichlorodiphenyltrichloroethane) was found in a pond. DDT enters the pond as runoff from farmland which has been sprayed with the insecticides.

  DDT increases or biomagnifies if we look at a food chain. DDT is fat-soluble, meaning animals store it in fatty tissues. It also takes a relatively long amount of time to break down.

Thus, if a predator consumes multiple organisms and each organism has a small amount of DDT, the amount of DDT in the predator is going to be the result of all of those small amounts combined.

In the given figure, we see that the concentration of DDT is increased at successive trophic levels, say if it starts at 0.003 ppb (ppb = parts per billion) in water, it can ultimately reach 25 ppm (ppm = parts per million) in fish eating birds, through biomagnifications.

High concentrations of DDT disturb calcium metabolism in birds, which causes thinning of eggshell and their premature breaking, eventually causing decline in bird populations.

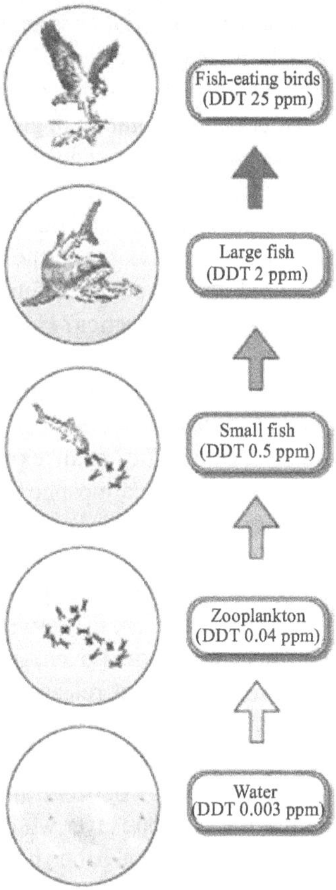

Fig.: Biomagnifications of DDT in an aquatic food chain

Note

Organisms at the top of the food chain are at a greater risk of damage due to biomagnifications. It is due to the reason that toxic elements cannot be absorbed and simultaneously they get transferred to the successive higher trophic levels resulting in more concentration of toxicants at the higher trophic level.

(c) Ground water depletion and replacement

- Ground water is generally considered to be safe and useful for drinking, agricultural and industrial purposes. Ground water is also less prone to pollution.
- However, in the recent years *ground water is depleting* due to the following reasons:
  - Its injudicious use both for agricultural and domestic purposes.
  - Deforestation also affects the level of ground water.
  - Lack of vegetation cover also results in very small amounts of water seeping through the ground.
  - An increase in water pollution is another factor that has reduced the availability of ground water.
- *Measures for replenishing ground water*:
  - Preventing over-exploitation of ground water.
  - Optimising water use and reducing water demand.
  - Rain water harvesting (RWH).
  - Preventing deforestation and plantation of more trees.
  - Rain water can be collected on the roof tops of buildings and can be stored underground for future use.

6. Why does ozone hole forms over Antarctica? How will enhanced ultraviolet radiation affect us?

Sol.

- Joseph Farman, Brian Gardiner, and Jonathan Shanklin discovered a recurring springtime Antarctic ozone hole in 1984.
- The ozone hole is formed due to an excessive use of increased concentration of chlorine in the atmosphere. A large amount of ODS (Ozone Depleting Substances) like CFCs (chlorofluorocarbons), N_2O, halons, SO_2, CH_4, Cl^- are released by advanced countries like USA, Japan, European countries. These are released in stratosphere, drift towards poles and reach there before the coming of winter. During winter (temp. 85°C) ice clouds are formed over Antarctica and no sunrise is received in polar areas. It catalyses release of Cl from CFCs. With the coming of spring season, the release of chlorine atoms causes the conversion of ozone into molecular oxygen. One atom of chlorine can destroy around 10,000 molecules of ozone and causes *ozone depletion*. All this leads to thinning of ozone layer which is more prominent over Antarctica region and called as the ozone hole. This hole disappears in summer due to free mixing of air of Antarctica with the rest of the global air.
- The formation of the ozone hole *will result on an increased concentration of UV-B radiations* on the Earth's surface.
- *Effects of enhanced UV Radiation* are as follows:

  (i) Snow blindness or inflammation of cornea.

  (ii) Damage of skin cells and development of skin cancer.

(iii) Damage to nucleic acids and proteins.
(iv) Reduced immunity.
(v) Higher number of cataracts in humans.

7. Discuss the role of women and communities in protection and conservation of forests.

Sol. Women and communities have played a major role in environmental conservation movements. It includes the following:

(i) *Amrita Bishnoi's wildlife protection project*

- This community strictly believes in the concept of simple living peacefully with nature.
- In 1731, to fulfill the order of king of Jodhpur for arranging wood for the construction of his new palace, minister and the workers went to Bishnoi village.

  Amrita Devi protested against king's men's attempt to cut trees as it was prohibited in Bishnoi religion. It was a party of Maharaja Abhay Singhji, Rular of Marwar (Jodhpur) state who wanted to fell green khejdali trees. Amrita Devi & her three daughter & more than 360 of other Bishnois lost their lives in saving trees & became martyers. This resistance by the people of the village forced the king to give up the idea of cutting trees.

(ii) *Chipko movement*

- This movement was started in 1974 in the village of Garhwal region of the Himalayas. In this movement, the women stopped the contractors from cutting forest trees by embracing them.
- Gaura Devi of village Gopeshwar in Chamoli district had led a movement, where in village people hugged the trees to save them from being cut.
- Many other people in different villages under the leadership of Chandi Prasad and Sunder Lal Bahuguna participated in similar protests.

8. What measures, as an individual, would you take to reduce environmental pollution?

Sol. Pollution prevention is any practice that reduces, eliminates, or prevents pollution at its source. It is also known as source reduction. It is a main global concern because of their harmful effects on a person's health and on the environment. Environmental pollution occurs in various forms, such as air pollution, water pollution, soil pollution, etc.

To reduce environmental pollution we should take following measures :

(i) Use of clean and renewable energy sources such as CNG and bio-fuels.
(ii) Reducing the use of fossil fuels and using catalytic converters in automobiles.
(iii) Optimising the use of water.
(iv) Using kitchen waste water in gardening and other household purposes.
(v) Composting of biodegradable kitchen waste.

(vi) Segregation of waste and composting of biodegradable kitchen waste.

(vii) Reducing the use of plastics and recycling and reuse of plastic and paper.

(viii) Disposing off waste safely.

(ix) Reducing use of polythene.

(x) Not disposing off waste in water bodies.

(xi) Making automobiles pollution free.

(xii) Prevention of noise pollution by using fire crackers/TV/musical instruments at permissible limits.

(xiii) Tree plantation in school, around residence.

9. Discuss briefly the following:

(a) Radioactive wastes

(b) Defunct ships and e-wastes

(c) Municipal solid wastes

Sol. (a) Radioactive waste

- *Radioactive waste* is usually a by-product of nuclear power generation and other applications of nuclear fission or nuclear technology, such as research and medicine.
- Nuclear waste is rich in radioactive materials that generate large quantities of ionising radiations such as gamma rays. These rays cause mutation in organisms, which often results in skin cancer. At high dosage, these rays can be lethal.
  Increased risk of cancer, birth defects & infertility are few harmful effects caused by nuclear waste. So, nuclear waste is an extremely potent pollutant.
- It was realised that the use of nuclear energy has two very serious inherent problems. The *first* is accidental leakage, as occurred in the Three Mile Island and Chernobyl incidents and the *second* is safe disposal of radioactive wastes. Safe disposal of radioactive wastes is a big challenge. It is recommended that nuclear wastes should be stored after pre-treatment in suitable shielded containers, which should then be buried in rocks.

(b) Defunct ships & e-wastes

- *Defunct ships*
  - These are dead ships of no longer in use. Such ships are broken down for scrap metal in countries such as India and Pakistan. Dismantling of defunct ship is a technically complex process, which is potentially harmful to the environment & human health.
  - These ships are a source of various toxicants such as asbestos, lead, mercury etc. Thus, they contribute to solid wastes that are hazardous to health.

  - The workers breaking the ships are not suitably protected and are exposed to toxic chemicals. The coastal areas in the vicinity of the ship-breaking yard also becomes polluted. At the international level, it is accepted that there is uncertainty about the relevant controls for the dismantling of such vessels & there is an urgent need to establish a specific enforceable control framework.
- *E-wastes or electronic wastes*
  - Electronic waste comprised of irrepairable computer and other electronic goods, generated by developed countries.
  - It is valuable source of secondary raw materials, if treated properly, however if not treated properly it is the major source of toxins.
  - These are rich in metals such as copper, iron, silicon, gold etc. These metals are highly toxic and pose serious health hazards.
  - People of developing countries are involved in the recycling process of these metals and therefore, get exposed to toxic substances present in these wastes.

  Eventually recycling is the only solution for the treatment of e-wastes provided it is carried out in an environment friendly manner.

(c) Municipal solid wastes
- These are commonly known as *trash or garbage*. It consists of everyday items such as product packaging, furniture, clothing, bottles, food scraps, newspapers. appliances, paints, batteries etc.
- The open dumps of municipal wastes serve as a breeding ground for flies, mosquitoes, and other disease-causing microbes. Hence, it is necessary to dispose municipal solid waste properly to prevent the spreading of diseases.
- Sanitary landfills and incineration are the methods for the safe disposal of solid wastes. Source reduction, recycling and compositing are several municipal social waste management practices.

10. What initiatives were taken for reducing vehicular air pollution in Delhi? Has air quality improved in Delhi?

Sol. Delhi has been categorised as the fourth most polluted city of the world in a list of 41 cities. Burning of fossil fuels has added to the pollution of air in Delhi.
- *Various steps which have been taken to improve the quality of air in Delhi* are as follows:
  - Introduction of CNG (Compressed Natural Gas): By the order of the supreme court of India, CNG-powered vehicles were introduced at the end of year 2006 to reduce the levels of pollution in Delhi. CNG is a clean fuel that produces very little unburnt particles.

- Phasing out of old vehicles.
- Introduction of green zones.
- Use of unleaded and low-sulphur petrol, and diesel.
- Use of catalytic converters in vehicles.
- Application of stringent pollution-level norms for vehicles.
- Implementation of Bharat stage I, which is equivalent to euro II norms in vehicles of major Indian cities.

• *Yes, air quality has been improved in Delhi.* The introduction of CNG-powered vehicles led to a substantial fall in the level of CO_2 and SO_2. However, the problem of suspended particulate matter (SPM) and respiratory suspended particulate matter (RSPM) still persists.

11. Discuss briefly the following :

(a) Greenhouse gases

(b) Catalytic converter

(c) Ultraviolet B

Sol. (a) Greenhouse gases

• The greenhouse effect refers to an overall increase in the average temperature of the Earth due to the presence of greenhouse gases.

• Many greenhouse gases occur naturally in the atmosphere, such as carbon dioxide, methane, water vapour, and nitrous oxide, while others are synthetic. Those that are man-made include the chlorofluorocarbons (CFCs), hydrofluorocarbons (HFCs) and Perfluorocarbons (PFCs), as well as sulfur hexafluoride (SF_6).

• These gases has the property of absorbing infrared radiation (net heat energy) emitted from Earth's surface and re-radiating it back to Earth's surface, thus contributing to the greenhouse effect. When solar radiations reach the Earth, some of these radiations are absorbed. These absorbed radiations are released back into the atmosphere which is then trapped by the greenhouse gases present in the atmosphere. This helps in keeping our planet warm and thus, helps in human survival.

• An increase in the amount of greenhouse gases can lead to an excessive increase in the Earth's temperature, thereby causing global warming.

Note

Carbon dioxide, methane, and water vapour are the most important greenhouse gases.

(b) Catalytic converter

- Catalytic converter are used to reduce emission of poisonous gases like nitrogen oxides, carbon monoxide & unreacted hydrocarbon in automotive emission.
- It is made of platinum, palladium and rhodium and is used as catalyst.
- As the vehicular discharge passes through the catalytic converter, the unburnt hydrocarbons present in it get converted into carbon dioxide and water. Carbon monoxide and nitric oxide released by catalytic converters are converted into carbon dioxide and nitrogen gas (respectively).
- The only precaution required is not to use gasoline having lead as lead inactivates the catalysts of the converter.

(c) Ultraviolet B

- Ultraviolet B is one of the three types of invisible light rays given off by the sun.
- Ultraviolet B penetrates the ozone layer in attenuated form & reaches Earth.
- It induces many health hazards in humans. UV–B damages DNA and activates the process of skin ageing. It also causes skin darkening and skin cancer. High levels of UV–B cause corneal cataract in human beings. It also reduce rate of photosynthesis in phytoplankton, diversity of aquatic ecosystem.